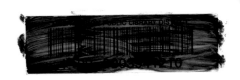

Can Mom Live Alone?

Can Mom Live Alone?

*Practical Advice on
Helping Aging Parents
Stay in Their Own Home*

by

Vivian F. Carlin, Ph.D.

Lexington Books

D.C. Heath and Company • Lexington, Massachusetts • Toronto

Library of Congress Cataloging-in-Publication Data

Carlin, Vivian F., 1919–
Can mom live alone?: practical advice on helping aging parents
stay in their own home / by Vivian F. Carlin.
p.   cm.
Includes bibliographical references and index.
ISBN 0-669-21735-2 (alk. paper)—ISBN 0-669-21736-0 (pbk. :
alk. paper)
1. Aged—Housing—United States.   2. Aged—Services for—United
States.   I. Title.
HD7287.92.U54C36   1991
649.8—dc20   90-25298
                                                              CIP

Published simultaneously in Canada
Printed in the United States of America
Casebound International Standard Book Number: 0–669–21739–2
Paperbound International Standard Book Number: 0–669–21736–0
Library of Congress Catalog Card Number: 90–25298

The paper used in this publication meets the minimum requirements of
American National Standard for Information Sciences—Permanence
of Paper for Printed Library Materials, ANSI Z39.48-1984. ∞™

Year and number of this printing:

91 92 93 94 95 8 7 6 5 4 3 2 1

*To my husband Benson
and my son Richard and his wife, Jessica, who
offered invaluable support and advice.*

Contents

Acknowledgments

I would like to thank the staff and participants at the following housing and community programs and social agencies who gave so generously of their time: American Homestead; Arkville, N.Y., Nutrition Site; Autumn Years; California Home Equity Conversion Coalition; Camden County (N.J.) Senior Center; COPSA; County of Somerset (N.J.) Office on Aging; Essex-Newark (N.J.) Legal Services, Senior Citizen Division; Highland Park (N.J.) Senior Center; HUD, Newark (N.J.) Office; Hudson County (N.J.) Office on Aging; Jeanes/Foulkeways Life-Care-at-Home Plan; Jewish Family Service of Delaware Valley; Mercer County (N.J.) County Office on Aging Outreach; Mercer County (N.J.) Legal Services Project for the Elderly; Mercer Street (N.J.) Friends Adult Day Care Center; National Association of Area Agencies on Aging; National Association of Private Geriatric Care Managers; New Jersey State Division on Aging; Older Adult Resources and Services (OARS); Phoenicia (N.Y.) Nutrition Site; Pine Hill (N.Y.) Social Club; Princeton (N.J.) Senior Resource Center; U.S. Department of Housing and Urban Development, Office of Policy Development and Research; Virginia Housing Development Authority; West Windsor (N.J.) Senior Citizen Center; Youth Employment Service of Princeton (N.J.) Intergovernmental Program.

In addition, I would like to thank family, friends, and many older people who shared their experiences with me. Their help was indispensable in the creation of this book which I hope will serve my readers well as a guide to making wise housing decisions.

An extra thanks to Terri Baker who did the special typing for me.

Introduction

Growing old today offers more possibilities for the good life than ever before, but it also brings with it some very tough decisions. After health, the most difficult of these involve housing. Often the former depends on the latter: where and how the elderly live can affect their well-being as much as what they eat. And living alone in old age can be hazardous to a person's health.[1]

Yet we know that the majority of the elderly not only live independently, but prefer to do so, and that there is as wide a range of ability, talent, and life-styles among the old as among the young. Aging only accentuates the individuality developed over a lifetime. Some common threads, however, do run through the aging process, becoming more predominant the older we get. Physical changes occur, such as hearing and vision losses, decreased muscle strength and agility, and increased sensitivity to extremes of heat and cold.[2]

Physical frailties, in turn, can and often do lead to negative psychological and social changes. The life circle, already reduced by retirement and the departure or loss of family members and friends, shrinks still further. Mobility is curtailed, and more and more time is spent in the home. A deteriorating neighborhood may aggravate fears for personal safety and increase the difficulties of shopping and socializing.[3]

Stories abound of lonely older people who become depressed and neglect themselves and their homes, disregarding even basic hygiene and nutrition. This often leads to cycles of illness and deepening despair. Depression in the elderly can be brought on by a personal illness or by the illness or death of a dear friend or close relative, by declining mobility, by becoming the victim of an accident or theft, by the adverse effects of medication, by poor nutrition, and so on.[4]

Until quite recently, senility was thought to be a normal part of the aging process. But recent research disproves this belief. We are learning that normal aging need not mean mental dysfunction. Such impairment can often be traced to a specific disease, to overmedication, to a nutritional deficiency, or even to depression.[5]

Much more needs to be learned about the aging process. Society was not prepared for the population explosion that has occurred among our top age groups: consequently much of the territory is still unexplored. More than 11 percent of the U.S. population is sixty-five years of age or older. Projections indicate that this percentage will increase in the next forty years until one in five people will be over sixty-five. This rapid increase will be caused by reduced infant mortality rates, declining birth rates, the aging of the baby boom population, and declining mortality rates for the elderly. In addition to the increased numbers and percentages of older people in our population, a greater number of the elderly will be living into their eighties and nineties. In ten years, those over seventy-five will constitute nearly half of the elderly population. In 1985, the United States census indicated that life expectancy at age sixty-five was 14.6 years for men and 18.7 years for women.[6]

Approximately 75 percent of the elderly own their own homes; 80 percent of these homes are mortgage-free. However, many of these houses were built years ago with no or inadequate insulation, making them more expensive to heat, cool, and maintain. In addition, some of the homes are structurally unsound or in need of major repairs.

A national task force on housing found that 47 percent of low-income homeowners were people over sixty-five and that their houses were more likely to be in poor condition than those belonging to other age groups. In addition, older renters were more disadvantaged than their younger counterparts since of all age groups they pay the highest proportion of their incomes for rent. According to a Harvard study, the average older woman who lives alone pays almost half of her income for rent.[7]

In spite of their homes' structural and economic disadvantages, most of the elderly prefer to remain living in their own homes. This preference for aging in place is consistent with the fact that in any one year only 9 percent of the elderly move as compared to 18 percent of the other age groups.[8]

The American Association of Retired Persons (AARP) conducted a national housing survey in 1989 and found that 86 percent of the elderly did not want to move from their present dwelling; this finding indicates a significant increase over the 78 percent of the elderly who expressed a desire to "stay put" in a similar study conducted in 1986.[9]

Since the overwhelming majority of older people want to continue living in their own homes, I felt that it was important to write a book that would help them fulfill this desire. *Can Mom Live Alone?* discusses the various housing programs, services, and agencies that are available to seniors to aid them in leading happier, healthier, and more comfortable lives.

This book stresses the need for planning, and especially planning before a crisis occurs. According to the AARP survey, more than half of the elderly have done no planning for their future housing needs; this percentage is even higher for those over seventy-five years of age. Those older people who are the most vulnerable are the ones least likely to evaluate what options exist and which ones would suit their needs.[10]

In most recent studies the seniors' decision to remain living at home was equated with their strong desire to maintain or increase their independence, privacy, and social relationships. Moreover, home ownership gives the elderly freedom and a sense of control over their own lives.

In chapter 1, I explore the meaning and importance of home for the elderly who want to remain living in their own homes. I discuss the fact that people's life experiences and memories are reflected in their homes. Also, home ownership ensures privacy, confers independence and greater ability to control one's own life, and manifests social status.

Being house-rich and cash-poor is a common situation for many elderly today. They have equity in homes that they bought many years earlier, but are struggling with a poor cash flow that hinders their ability to remain in and maintain the upkeep and repairs on their houses. Programs aimed at resolving these problems such as home equity conversion or property tax deferral are described in detail in chapter 2.

Loneliness is an increasing problem for the elderly, particularly for those who live alone. Nearly one-third of the older population lives alone. These are usually widows over seventy-five. In the next thirty years the 8.5 million elderly people who are living alone today are expected to increase in number to 13.3 million. Some of the most frail and vulnerable elderly live alone. The older one is, the more likely that he or she will be living alone.[11] This group also has the highest percentage of those who are lonely. This loneliness problem is exacerbated by the fact that we live in a highly mobile society so that many adult children no longer live close enough to their older parents to supply "hands-on" support. In chapter 3, I present possible solutions, such as home sharing and creating accessory apartments.

As I mentioned earlier, many elderly homeowners live in old houses that are badly in need of repair. They are unable to afford the maintenance costs and/or can not cope with the hiring and the overseeing of the repairmen. Chapter 4 describes programs that provide carpentry, plumbing, masonry work, painting, roofing repairs, window replacement, and winterization services for the elderly. Maintenance services, such as Mr. Fixit, and chore services are also discussed.

More accidents occur in the home than any other place. The elderly are particularly vulnerable to home accidents. But looking about with a critical eye and making small changes can make the family home safer and more comfortable for aging residents. Suggestions for remodeling to create a downstairs bathroom and bedroom, rearranging furniture, installing safety grab bars, illuminating floor thresholds and stairs, lowering cabinets, purchasing nightlights, adding plastic chairs in the tub/shower, and switching to European hand-held showers are among the many ideas presented.

Many older people and their families do not know about existing services and programs. And even if they do, many are unlikely to use these services because they equate them with "welfare" or feel that it makes them seem more dependent or of a lower status. This situation is most unfortunate since sometimes all an older person needs to remain independent is to be able to use some community resources to help him or her resolve financial, physical, or psychological problems. Chapter 6 describes local services and programs such as senior centers, nutrition sites, adult day-care centers, friendly visitor, telephone reassurance, and legal aid.

Knowing that there is a place where one can turn in times of trouble to secure help with problems can often make a vast difference to the elderly's sense of well-being. Chapter 7 discusses the information and referral services offered by many states and most area agencies on aging. Typical problems presented to these agencies and solutions offered to people requesting assistance on the telephone or in person are discussed in detail. Other resources such as family service agencies, mental health centers, and geriatric care managers are also described.

Chapter 8 discusses a number of older couples who wanted to remain in their own homes but found the northern climate too difficult and have therefore relocated to the South. Most of them are very satisfied with this move and find to their pleasant surprise that living in a southern state has other advantages besides a warmer climate. The chapter also includes some caveats to be considered before one considers making such a move.

Although this book is basically geared to giving information to those older people who want to "stay put," a time may come when living at home is no longer a viable solution. Other housing alternatives may need to be considered and a move planned. Chapter 9 presents a brief summary of the various housing options available to the elderly.

Chapter 10 summarizes the material presented in chapters 2 through 8, evaluates the pros and cons of the major alternatives, and presents several self-questionnaires to help older people select the most suitable option(s).

I end the book with a look to the future where I discuss trends in housing services, and describe a number of new pilot programs to help seniors remain at home. In addition, this last chapter summarizes information about the community agencies that can offer the elderly help in solving their housing problems.

This book presents anecdotal material based on real people living in real situations to illustrate how some of the elderly's housing problems were solved through the use of different community resources. My book is enriched by the voices of the elderly themselves, who talk about their lives, state their opinions, and describe their feelings. I have fictionalized the names of my sources to protect their privacy. I hope that my readers will be able to identify with some of the stories and find the information helpful for themselves or their older relatives.

No Place Like Home

The Meaning and Importance of Home for Older People

A large majority of older people prefer to remain in their own homes. Why do they consider this so important? What does the home mean to them? And what does leaving that home and moving to another living arrangement mean?

Ed and Beth were staying with their mother, Eileen McNeil. Her husband, their father, had just died and they had come to help her put her affairs in order. Ed, an accountant, was reviewing all her finances, while Beth was helping her mother go through some of her husband's clothing and papers. Although Ed and Beth were still grieving over the sudden death of their father, they were very concerned about their mother's physical and emotional health and wanted to give her as much support as possible. The McNeils had always been a close-knit family and Ed and Beth were quite ready to rise to this occasion.

Eileen was sixty-five years old and had had diabetes for five years. More recently, she had had a heart attack, and although it was a fairly mild one, now that she was going to be living alone, Ed and Beth were concerned about what would happen if she had a second attack. "Mother," Ed said, "I don't want to rush you but I think it's very important that you think about where you will live now that dad is gone."

"Why," Eileen replied, "I plan to continue to live in this house as I have done for the past thirty years. This is my home and I think your father would have wanted me to stay here."

"But who will mow the lawn, and take care of the garden, and do all the repairs that dad did?" asked Beth. Eileen's house was situated on a relatively small, but intensively cultivated, lot. It was a split-level with a finished playroom, laundry room, and powder room in the basement, a living room-dining room, eat-in kitchen, and large screened-in porch on the first level, and three bedrooms and a bath on the upper level.

Eileen started to become very agitated at her children's questions, so Ed and Beth both realized that they should stop this discussion now but continue it, very gently, on another occasion. About a month later, Ed and Beth raised the subject of their mother moving in with Beth. This time she seemed a littler calmer and was more receptive to the topic of change. However, she made it quite clear that she felt she could take care of herself and would not consider moving in with either of them. Eileen said, "Remember when you were both little and grandma moved in with us? She slept in the small spare room and shared our bath? You both complained a lot at that time and weren't very happy with that arrangement, and I must say that I couldn't blame you. Well, I don't want to be in that situation. And I think you'd agree, wouldn't you?" Beth replied that they did not expect Eileen to move in with either of them but hoped instead that they could find her an apartment close by one of them. However, that alternative was not appealing to their mother since she did not want to move to a place where she did not know anyone. Eileen said, "You remember my old friend, Mary? Well, she recently moved close to her daughter and found that she missed all her old friends, and didn't know anyone but her daughter and her family. Mary became very unhappy because she found herself becoming too dependent on her daughter and her son-in-law."

Beth and Ed understood their mother's fears but asked her to reconsider. Eileen reluctantly agreed to let them look for an acceptable apartment for her, but would not promise anything more than that.

A few weeks later, Ed found a very attractive four-room apartment not far from his house. It had two bedrooms and one and a half baths and he thought it was perfect for his mother. He shared this news with his sister before telling Eileen, and the two planned their strategy. Their mother kept her word, and drove down to her son's house for the weekend. Ed took her to the apartment but acted very nonchalant and did not apply any pressure. He was very proud of his cool approach and allowed his mother plenty of time to look over the apartment.

"It's very nice," she said, "But where would I put all my beautiful furniture—grandma's old chest and dining room set—and all the paintings dad and I have collected over the years?" It became apparent that nothing Ed could say would change her mind, and so they decided to drive back to his house and continue the discussion about his mother's future housing plans.

Ed asked his mother how she planned to handle snow shoveling and carrying the heavy trash barrels from the garage to the curb for rubbish collection every week. And Beth raised the issue of her mother being constantly reminded of her husband if she continued to live in their house. Beth continued, "And wouldn't it be better for you mom if you moved away from all the sad memories and built a new life for yourself?"

This last question was just too much for Eileen to bear and she really exploded. "You children just don't understand, it's not sad, but comforting for me to stay in this house where I have such wonderful memories of your father! And I know my grocer, my banker, my pharmacist, and have so many good friends in this town. I love all the volunteer work that I do here at my church, and at all the fairs and other fund-raising activities." She began to become quite rhapsodic about her life and went on to describe how much her bimonthly trips to the neighboring metropolitan area, where she visited the museums and went to the theater, meant to her.

Eileen continued to share some of her thoughts with Ed and Beth about how much her home meant to her. "I've never told you this before, but I feel much more confident with people I've known for a long time and I'm rather uncomfortable with new people. And I do have loads of old friends here. My house represents stability to me. It is predictable and makes me feel more in control of my own life. This house gives me the strength to face life alone without your father."

Beth and Ed began to realize just how attached their mother was to the house she had shared with their father for so many years, and began to understand why she could not and would not give up this home, at least for the time being. However, Beth wanted to share one more concern with her mother, and so she asked her what she would do if her health deteriorated and she was not able to manage alone. Eileen responded, "I can hire someone to take care of me. No, better yet, we would share my house and she would become like a family member. In this way, I could continue to have control of what I eat and even to do some of the cooking if I am able to. And I love being able to entertain family and friends. If I gave up this house how could you and your families spend weekends and holidays with me?"

Eileen's resolve not to move typified the attitude of the participants in this study, almost all of whom shared a strong desire to continue living in their own home. As one elderly lady said, "They will have to carry me out in a basket—I *won't* give up this house while I'm alive!" Another said, "As long as I can afford it, I won't move. Having your own home is the greatest blessing from the Lord."

The reasons people gave for staying put were many and varied, but two important ones, as Eileen has already suggested, were maintaining independence and control over their own lives. One gentleman told me that when you have your own place, "No one tells you what to do. You can do whatever you like. You can be independent. I can walk around in my house with no clothes on if I want to." An older woman put it a little differently: "No one is going to tell me what to do, what I can eat. If I don't want to clean, I don't have to. When you're older it's the first time you're free of kids and other responsibilities." This sense of control and feeling of independence that is associated with home ownership appears to be very important in counteracting negative feelings arising from lack of control over the physical changes that accompany the aging process.

Implicit in some of the above remarks is the fact that their own home provides them with a sense of privacy. "I like to be alone and have my privacy. I don't want to be with a bunch of people all the time. Privacy is a million dollars," one person told me. Another put it this way: "I wouldn't like eating all my meals every day with other people, and I don't want to be forced to participate in organized activities."

To be able to continue following their own life-styles is another important reason for remaining in the home. "I love gardening and want to be able to have a garden," said one of my informants. Another said, "My big house means that I can continue to entertain my family and friends, and this is very important to me." The home provides some people with the opportunity to pursue favorite hobbies. One widow said, "My house gives me the space I need for all my collectibles." A former professor continued to do research and needed to refer to his enormous collection of books—a collection he could never transfer to an apartment. A third person worked with tools and enjoyed building patios and small accessory buildings.

Home is a known quantity, familiar and loved, associated with life history and fond memories. Older people told me, "I enjoy my home. It gives me pleasure. My furniture, decorations, and collectibles are very meaningful to me. My house is a link to my husband and my children since I have many of their possessions on the walls and in the rooms and I see them every day. If I had to move I couldn't keep these things that are so important to me."

A home represents many different things to different people, as the following statements indicate: "My home makes me very happy and content"; "It gives me so many more things to do"; "I have a paid-up mortgage and it's cheaper to stay put"; "My home gives me the self-assurance to do what I always wanted to do"; "Your own home gives you a challenge and keeps you in good physical and mental shape"; "When I put the key in the door, I get a special feeling that this is mine"; "Having your own home makes the difference between being happy or just existing and waiting for the day you die." As these comments indicate, home ownership contributes significantly to maintaining positive feelings about life as one ages. The importance of one's own home extends beyond the actual house itself. It includes familiarity with the neighborhood, its stores and services, having neighbors one knows and trusts, and being close to children and friends. One of the more interesting aspects of the meaning of home was seldom articulated directly but often implicit in the comments people made: the home represented an extension of one's self, or one's self-identity. A widow in her early seventies, still working in a professional capacity, indicated this connection between home and self-image when she said: "My home illustrates my life and who I think I am. My paintings, my books, medals, testimonials, furnishings—all say who I am. This house shows all the ages and stages I've been through, it testifies to my past existence. It is my personality. The more remote I become from the active 'me' the more I need this house to testify to my former active self I took pride in—as contrasted with the frail person I fear I may become."

I spoke with this widow at another time, after she had thought more about what her home meant to her. Now she was even more articulate:

> You ask why I want to remain in my home when there are sensible alternative arrangements available. Logically, a ten-room, four-bathroom house is unsuitable for a seventy-one-year-old woman who lives alone, and I should condense into something smaller. A three-room apartment is often suggested, and some think a studio would be enough for my needs. That advice comes from a narrowly functional view, a kitchen to cook and eat in, a bedroom to sleep in, a bathroom for bathing and toileting, and maybe a room to entertain guests. But on thinking it over, I realize that my home meets other, more subtle needs. The older I get and the further removed from my energetic accomplished middle-aged self, the more I need this home as a testament to the person I was during the active stage of my life. The family portraits in my bathroom show a three-year-old me among the chickens on my grandmother's farm, a bride and groom, the mother with young children, a widow, still energetic and finding a new career, and then the grandchildren and in-laws. The paintings and sculpture in other rooms bespeak art interests and sensitivity to beauty. The soft chairs invite friends to have tea and gossip with me. Art deco objects and a Christmas keepsake collection of books and cards represent a hobby, a collection that grew over the years. The garden is overfilled with plants, and even rocks that I gathered in this place and that remind me of past trips. There are little sprigs that grew into big bushes and little seedlings that are now trees two and three stories high.
>
> What will I be at the end of my life, in that studio apartment or retirement home? A thin, pale, wrinkled, gray-haired anonymous crone. Maybe I will be friends with some other crones, but what young person will want to visit me for any reasons other than duty or compassion? I often have young people or middle-aged people visiting now—they love to look around and see the things I gathered 'round me over the years. They get ideas for their own home furnishings, they look forward to experiencing and collecting as I did, and they enjoy a tea party with my old-fashioned dishes and cloths. It is fun to entertain a cousin's child or a friend's child, show off the crowded house full of interesting

clutter, give them a momento—a book, a painting, something from my life of gatherings—and send them happily on their way.

If I am lucky, I can live this way until I die. And if it is a choice of living an extra few years in a constricted environment or staying on here as long as I can, I am going to try to stay here. Home, sweet home! a phrase with a lot of meaning for me!

Only a few studies on this aspect of the meaning of home have been conducted, but I found an excellent one in the *Journal of Gerontology: Social Sciences* written by Robert L. Rubenstein. He described how older people view their homes and their homes' contents as an extension of themselves. He obtained his information by conducting interviews with a group of informants that he returned to regularly over a period of time. In general, he found that the furnishings and other articles in the house were endowed with important personal meaning for each individual. By way of illustration he cites excerpts from some of his interviews. The following are stories of three elderly widows, adapted from his article.[1]

Mrs. Stein has lived in her small row house for most of her seventy-six years. Many important life events took place in its confines, shared over time with her parents, husband, siblings, and children. She was a person who amply and intently illustrated her life through environmental features. In addition to the meaning-laden photos and furniture, she had some twenty or so small plastic and ceramic objects: figurines, bric-a-brac, and animal sculptures. . . . She noted that, "I like them." . . . She did not express much intense emotional involvement with these objects, but they marked and filled her space, gave her sensory pleasure, had a story, and gave her stories to tell, and added texture to her rooms.

A much more important involvement with her house came out in a later interview when Mrs. Stein said that

she felt as if she was part of her house and it was part of her. She noted one time: "It's a crazy thing to say, but I love it here. I love the feel of this house. I love being in it. And I think if I had to be put away somewhere, who knows, I think I'd want to die. But I enjoy being here. I feel all the presences of all the things that ever happened to me. Right here. Even though I don't get to see my mother and my father, visually; sometimes in my dreams, but most of the time I feel their presence, their comfort, their warmth. It's ridiculous, but that's how I feel about it. Maybe my children can't understand that you can love a house. Love has many, many definitions. . . . I feel all my thoughts and all my prayers and all my wishes and all my trials and tribulations were settled right here in this house."

Rubenstein felt that this was a remarkable account. Mrs. Stein's statements clearly indicate how a house can have a positive psychological effect on people. A house is not merely an important physical place. In Mrs. Stein's case, her home embodies her past; it functions as part of her and carries with it all her important values and life experiences: "She went on to say . . . that when she feels unwell, she feels better at home; she noted that she's taken care of the house and it in turn takes care of her."

Another interesting person Rubenstein encountered was Mrs. Collins.

Among her possessions were two fine tables dating from the mid-eighteenth century. They were lovingly maintained and centrally displayed. The tables came to her through her husband's mother and her husband, and were each destined to go to one of her two sons. Both Mrs. Collins and her husband came from "society." Her father, an alcoholic, lost his money and the family's circumstances were greatly reduced. Much of our conversation focused on Mrs. Collins' relationship with her husband, his severe alcoholism, their terrible marriage and its dissolution, his hospitalization, the negative effects of these events on her and her children, her husband's death, and her struggles since then including cancer and her awareness that the doctor felt she had a limited time to live. Yet she was a tough person who persevered. Indeed, despite her poor relationship with her husband and her frequent unhappiness, she held on to these tables not only as lovely objects, but, she noted, as representations of where she had come from, what she had aspired to, and to a great extent, who she still felt herself to be, inside, despite the difference between her actual circumstances and her ideal. The tables stood, to her, for continuity, class values, and the life-style to which she aspired, that she had once attained, and which, she felt, she partially maintained through the keeping of her values. Thus, besides their display value as decoration, they were emblematic of a variety of key meanings and themes in her life.

Mrs. Stein, in a later interview, described the activities that she did in her home. She mentioned

performing household tasks, such as sweeping up, dusting, replacing moved objects, and picking up newspapers, casually, with no prior planning and as her health dictated. To her this is a conscious, named procedure in which, as she described it, she becomes attuned to what should be done in her house and, at the same time, the restrictions her body places on doing these things. An important accompaniment is a feeling of being a part of, or "with" the house, and an important meaning that she articulated was continuity, doing it as she had always done it.

She also described her routine activity of playing solitaire. Its stated purpose was to pass the time. Yet it also admittedly served as a background activity, something repetitive to occupy the hands and part of the mind, which provided the opportunity for pleasurable reminiscence. Mrs. Berg reported that she spent much of her afternoons at her kitchen table playing solitaire, listening to music on the radio, monitoring the food she was cooking, and reminiscing. As she noted, features of the home would "get me to thinking." In this way, she again became "with" her home as its features could provide objects and settings for thought.

I have been exploring the meaning of home, particularly for those older people who have lived in the same place for most of their adult life. I have discovered that one's own home is a familiar and known quantity, and is viewed as an extension of oneself. A home is situated in a specific neighborhood, where neighbors, friends, shopping and other services have been a consistent part of one's life. Family, a vital source of love and support, may live close by. The home is a source of fond memories about meaningful aspects of one's life: spouse, children, family gatherings, and other pleasant things. A home gives one a sense of competence and security, because the older homeowner has learned through experience how to manage and cope with his or her familiar environment. Remaining in one's own home can represent higher status, since in our society home ownership indicates that a person is more independent, and hence more worthy. A house often represents an older person's only or largest asset, but the owner usually has good reasons to resist exchanging his or her home for mere financial security; often no amount of money can compensate the owner for the memories and other intangible values he or she must sacrifice when giving up a cherished home.

In addition to the positive and important meanings people associate with their homes, many people remain where they are for the simple, practical reason that making a significant change is difficult at any stage of life, but becomes more difficult when one is older. Physical and emotional stress usually occur whenever one changes one's place of residence, and such stress can be more pronounced in the elderly. In addition to the stress accompanying the actual move, more stress is produced by the need to adjust to and cope with the new living situation. The double stress of leaving an old, familiar place and readjusting to a new and strange place can be particularly devastating to the elderly.

Some people stay put because even considering a move provokes a fear of the unknown. Change produces anxiety because one does not know what to expect; staying put, whatever the disadvantages, at least provides the comfort of the known. Changing one's present housing also usually means exchanging a larger living space for a smaller living space. Thus, the older person has to decide which possessions and furnishings to keep and which to dispose of. A reduction in the scale of living space generates real problems that can have an adverse emotional impact. A move that means coping with a smaller kitchen, for example, can hurt a woman who has always taken pride in her abilities as a cook and hostess, just as the loss of his cellar workshop can be a serious blow to the pride of an amateur craftsman.

Our culture encourages older persons to stay in their own homes because of the positive value it places on economic independence. Moving often implies a loss of status and control, especially when a different living arrangement is equated with an institution. Moving to another type of housing is thought of as an admission that one is getting older and needs a more protected environment and more supportive services. This again can have negative connotations. And lastly, leaving one's home can be associated with death and dying.

Because most people do want to continue living in their own homes, it is important to review briefly the changes that accompany aging that may make this difficult if one doesn't plan ahead. There can be changes in the family structure: a spouse can become very ill or die, for example, and children or close friends can move away. These changes adversely affect one's informal support system. There can be changes in the ability to pay for the maintenance, taxes, and upkeep of the home: inflation can erode one's purchasing power, housing costs can rise very rapidly, medical expenses can become overwhelming—to name just a few common occurrences that can have a negative impact on one's ability to afford keeping one's home.

There are also physical changes that accompany aging. Older people experience losses in functional ability. Impaired hearing and sight, and chronic conditions such as heart problems and arthritis may make it difficult to move about in the home; acts that one used to take for granted such as climbing stairs or using the bathtub now become difficult or even impossible. Physical changes increase the possibilities for accidents in the home. These changes also create a more restricted social world due to the limitations in mobility and the inability to continue driving a car. A shrinking arena for activity and social relations can quickly increase feelings of isolation and loneliness.

Unfortunately, many older people either assume that there will be no real changes in their lives, or recognize that change is inevitable but choose to put off preparing for change until it is too late. One such person who has made no plans for continuing to remain in her own house is a woman I shall call Susan Beech. Ms. Beech is 86 and has been a widow for nine years. Her husband had been in state government and retired 20 years ago. However, he continued to write books on government and related subjects. Unfortunately, he developed congestive heart failure five years before he died and was ill on and off during that time. They had two children, a son and a daughter. The daughter lives in a neighboring state, about one hundred miles away, and the son lives close by, in the next town.

Although Susan and her husband had lived in the same community all of their married life, they did not move into their present house until 1960. It is a seven-room ranch with an unfinished basement. Both Susan and her husband had advanced degrees. And, although Susan did very little paid work outside the home, she did work with her husband on his books and together they produced over a dozen. Susan enjoyed working with her husband. He, in turn, needed her collaboration since his eyesight was poor. She did most of the library research. She confessed that after her husband died, she did try to write alone, but that this just did not work out.

Susan is a slim, attractive, and extremely intelligent woman who has always been very active in her community. She still drives a car, walks with a spritely gait, and appears much younger than her years. She has not had any serious physical problems and continues to enjoy relatively good health for a person of her age. Although she still gardens, she has curtailed her vegetable and flower gardens and has hired someone to do the heavy outdoor work.

Aside from raising two children and helping her husband write a number of books, she was very active in several women's organizations, serving as a chairman and president of the local group and a member of the state chapter. She served on the PTA and the adult school board, and organized a local branch of the American Field Service. She was appointed to the municipal health department, served on the regional health commission, and became chairperson of the regional board of health. As if this were not enough for one person, she was one of the founders of the Council of Community Services and served as its president for two terms. Presently, Susan is still a member of this council and the regional health commission, and serves as the liason to the Joint Commission on Aging. Still actively involved, she rarely misses any meetings.

In addition to her community activities, she enjoys being at home where she reads murder mysteries, nonfiction books on the environment, and the daily newspapers. She watches TV, and is particularly fond of nature programs. Susan has a large dog and she walks the dog twice a day. She also takes nature walks and does some bird watching. She drives to her daughter's house, two hours away, about once every two months. This past year she spent much of the time preparing a family history and wrote a very detailed account complete with several elaborate family trees and photographs. Susan Xeroxed copies for each family member and organized a large reunion on the West coast where all of her sisters and their families reside. She was very proud of this accomplishment, an outstanding family success.

Susan does not expect to have to move from her house. She told me:

> I enjoy living alone. I have many friends in the community that I see often and my son and his family live close by. I lead a good life. My whole life is built into this house—the garden, the dog, my neighbors—the house is a part of me. We built and designed this house and picked the location so that we backed up on a large wooded area. I have a real attachment to the grounds as well as the house, since we planted all the trees and have watched them grow along with our own children. I know all the birds that live in our yard and feel that they too are part of my past and present. If I ever have to give up my house I will feel as if I have lost part of myself. Also, I would find it most difficult to part with my possessions, particularly those meaningful family ones.

I have recounted Susan's story because she is typical of an educated, active elderly person who lives alone in a moderately large house and is not facing the possibility of changes in her functional abilities, although continuing to live in her own home is of paramount importance to her. Even though Susan has been fortunate to have reached the age of eighty-six in good health and is able to live in her usual life-style, she probably will not continue to be so lucky for the rest of her life. Since she has not considered any changes in her present living arrangement, let me do this for her by exploring what some of her options might be. I will describe what other older people have done to enable them to remain in their own homes.

House-Rich, Cash-Poor

Home Equity Conversion Plans,
Including Reverse Mortgages

A large majority of older people own their own homes and over 80 percent have paid off their mortgages. For many, their home is their only or largest asset. However, this money cannot be realized until the house is sold. For some of the elderly who want to remain in their homes but need added income for maintenance, medical expenses, or other financial needs, a new program called Home Equity Conversion (HEC) is now available through some banks, mortgage companies, and nonprofit agencies. This plan lets you turn part of the value of your home into cash without having to sell the house or repay a loan each month. Unfortunately, this program is available only in a limited number of areas. But this situation is changing rapidly, particularly since the federal government has recently developed an insured program (this program will be discussed later in the chapter).

HEC plans can be categorized according to the types of benefits they provide. In most plans, the cash received can be used for any purpose the homeowner chooses. Some plans do, however, dictate that the money must be used in a specific way, such as for making home repairs or paying property taxes. These special purpose loans are usually sponsored by the government. Plans also differ in the number of years during which benefits are provided: some are for a specific period of time, while others are for life. Some HEC loans provide for regular monthly payments, while others give the borrower an initial lump sum or allow for occasional withdrawals over the life of the loan.

HEC plans differ in two important ways. In some plans, the older person simply borrows against the equity in the home. In other plans, the home is actually sold but the former owner stays on under a leasing arrangement (sale leaseback). The former are the more usual and exist in two basic forms: (1) special purpose loans, and (2) reverse mortgages.

Before HEC loans became available, banks offered and still offer home equity loans and home equity lines of credit. These differ from the HEC plans I have been discussing because they require monthly repayments of the money loaned plus interest. The bank can foreclose and the borrower can lose his or her house if these payments are not made. HEC loans defer payments until the expiration of the loan term or the death of the homeowner.[1]

Special Purpose Loans

Deferred Payment Loans

The special purpose loans have been the most widely used HEC plans. The first type, called a deferred payment loan, can be used to repair or improve the home. These loans usually have a very low or no interest rate, and the loan does not have to be repaid until the death of the borrower or the sale of his or her house. The cash that the elderly homeowner receives can be used to improve or repair the house and make it more safe, or more accessible, or more energy-efficient. These loans are usually offered by local government agencies, but may not be available in all areas. Also, eligibility can be limited by income or assets criteria.[2]

Karen Roth had a widowed mother who was in her mid-eighties and continued to live alone in an isolated, ramshackle farmhouse. Two older brothers had died, and only Karen and a younger brother remained; he lived in a neighboring state. In recent years, Karen, who divorced her husband many years before, had considered moving back to the farm. But that would have meant a one and one-half hour drive each way to get to her job. Her friends dissuaded her, and she compromised by sleeping at the farmhouse one night a week and on weekends.

"I don't really mind," she said. "There's something comforting about sleeping in my old bed, especially now that I have had the roof fixed and I don't have to worry about it falling in on me. I enjoy the quiet, the birds, all the country things after a week of hustle 'n bustle. And momma's always glad to see me. She tells me a hundred times how nice it is to have me here."

Her friends wondered why Karen did not persuade her mother to sell the old house and move to a city apartment near Karen. "Even if she agreed to do it, I think it'd kill her," Karen answered. "Remember, she was born in that house. It belonged to her parents. My daddy moved in when they married. She's always telling me, 'I was born in this house and I mean to die here.' But I do worry about her, living alone out there. Even though I call her every day and she can reach me, what'd happen if she got sick and couldn't get to the phone?"[3]

A suggestion by a friend in the construction business triggered an idea to convert the upstairs of the farmhouse into a separate apartment. "More and more companies are putting up plants along the highway, and there's a big demand for housing out there already. We could rent the apartment to a young person or family, maybe lower the rent in exchange for them doing some chores around the house. Then it won't be so lonely out there for momma," Karen said.

A call to the county planning office established that there were no zoning restrictions in that rural location. But Karen was advised to get health department approval of the well and septic system before starting the renovation. Next, Karen discussed the idea with her mother, who had no objections, placing implicit faith in her daughter's judgment. When Karen warned her mother about the noise and dirt of construction, her mother was unconcerned. "I don't mind, Honey, because when it's over, we'll have something real fine. This house could use a lot of fixing!"

The big stumbling block was money. Karen had always found it difficult to accumulate any savings. After paying college costs for two of her children and investing in a few business ventures of the third, she had tried to start a new nest egg, only to deplete it on the desperately needed roof for the farmhouse. Again, her friend in construction came to the rescue, informing her of a county housing coalition that offered deferred payment loans to needy elderly homeowners.

Applying for this loan in her mother's name, Karen learned that it need not be paid back until the borrower died or sold the house, at which time the loan would have to be repaid by the heir or by the proceeds from the sale. Since Karen knew she would inherit the house, she understood that she would be responsible for repayment of the loan at some future date. She wondered whether this was the best method for financing the renovation and reviewed other HEC plans with her lawyer.

Karen and her mother rejected reverse mortgages and sale lease-backs, since in the former case they could not get a large enough lump sum to finance the apartment renovation and in the latter case Karen did not have the down payment needed for a sale leaseback. Both Karen and her mother finally agreed that a deferred payment loan would best accomplish their aims. Though the loan would place a lien on the property, it would also result in improvement to the house and conversion of underutilized space to produce income, thus increasing the property's value. And since the loan originated from a nonprofit group with interest set far below the market rate, Karen felt she could manage the payments without undue hardship when she became the owner.

"It's going to be great," she told her friends after the loan request had been granted and the construction blueprints drawn. "You know how much I love that old place. Now momma can have company out there and in five or six years, when I retire, I'll move out there into a nice, new apartment." Then she added, "Maybe, when I'm as old as momma, one of my children or grandchildren will come home to live with me."[4]

Property Tax Deferral Loans

The second type of HEC loan provides property tax deferral. Many elderly people living on fixed or shrinking incomes have difficulty paying their property taxes and thus risk losing their homes. To help them, government agencies advance the money needed to pay local property taxes in exchange for future repayment. The homeowner does not have to repay the loan unless he or she sells the house; if the house is not sold during the borrower's lifetime, his or her heirs pay back the loan after they inherit—if necessary by selling the property. In effect, the government is lending older people their tax money each year that they continue to live in their homes. Most tax deferral loans require a minimum age of sixty-five for recipients, and also an income below a certain level, although some states do not have any income limits.

Unfortunately, this very useful and successful program is available in only about one-third of the states. It is available in California, Colorado, Georgia, Illinois, Oregon, Texas, Utah, Washington, and Wisconsin, and in a few other states on a more limited basis.[5]

Reverse Mortgages

The reverse mortgage (RM) is the most flexible type of HEC. It works much like a standard mortgage loan, only in reverse. With an RM, the person retains ownership of the home, but at the same time some of the equity is converted into money for the homeowner's use. Eligibility for an RM requires that the home is owned free and clear of any mortgage, or nearly so. The house must be appraised for a specific value. This loan is paid to the homeowner in monthly installments either for life or over a specific number of years. The loan does not have to be paid back until the loan term is over. At that time, loan advances plus accrued interest must be repaid.

Although there are several different kinds of RMs, all share some common characteristics. First, because an RM is not paid back until some future time, the loan balance grows at an ever-increasing rate. Second, the amount of the monthly loan advance is dependent on the value of home equity, the interest rate on the loan, and the length of the loan term. In general, the more equity one has, the greater the potential size of the loan. On the other hand, the amount the borrower receives becomes smaller as the interest rate increases or the loan term becomes longer. Third, one can generally obtain an initial lump sum combined with smaller subsequent monthly payments.

Fourth, when the homeowner dies or when the house is sold, all RMs become due. A fifth feature common to most RMs is that repayment of the loan is limited by the value of the house: the lender cannot touch assets other than the house itself. The homeowner retains title to the house; the lender never owns it during the loan period. Most RMs permit one to repay the loan at any time without penalty. The elderly homeowner decides the amount of equity that needs to be turned into cash and how much needs to be reserved for other uses or for the estate. In addition, no restrictions are placed on how the money can be used. An RM usually provides the homeowner with more money than either a deferred payment loan or a tax deferral loan.

The money received from an RM is nontaxable and does not affect Social Security or Medicare benefits. Supplemental Security Income (SSI) or Medicaid are not affected as long as the cash is spent within the month the loan is received.[6]

RMs come in a variety of forms. The first type of RM is called a fixed-term or short-term loan. It provides monthly loan payments during a period of no less than three and no more than twelve years. When the term of the loan is over, the amount of the loan plus the accrued interest becomes due. A variation is called a split-term RM; this form also provides loans for a fixed period of time, but allows deferral of repayment of the loan until the person sells the house or dies.[7]

California offers a good example of a fixed-term RM program. Sponsored by the Independent Living Resource Center, the program is available in only certain counties. Participating lenders allow eligible seniors to borrow money at a fixed rate against their home— if it is clear of debt—for a term of three to twelve years.

The California program seems most suitable for frail elders looking for short-term income to assist them in living out their remaining years in their own home. Experience shows that most borrowers utilize these funds for live-in home care.

Mr. and Mrs. Davies were both in their late 80s when they applied for an RM loan. They were in need of a 24-hour live-in caretaker but had used up all their savings. A counselor met with them and their family and put them in touch with a medical and in-home supportive services program that is based on financial and health-care needs. This first step saved them the $300 per quarter they were paying for insurance, and in addition they received $1,500 per month toward home care. Since they still had a shortfall, it was decided to help them secure a five-year fixed-term RM. The maximum loan amount at that time was $125,000, which at an interest rate of 10.5 percent generated a $1,500 monthly income. Mr.

Davies died in his home 13 months after the loan closed, and Mrs. Davies was moved to a nursing home three years later. The house was then sold for $315,000. By then the amount due on the loan was $69,000, leaving Mrs. Davies with a net of $246,000.

The California loan program can also be utilized by younger, healthier seniors who want to "buy time" in the home. Mrs. Valez is eighty-one and in excellent health. She expects to live a long time because both her parents lived into their nineties. Her sister and she resided in the family home for twenty years after her husband died. Her sister recently passed away, and Mrs. Valez does not want to remain alone in the large five-bedroom house.

Mrs. Valez shopped around for a retirement center that fit her needs and found one she liked in a neighboring town. The center is under construction and will not be ready for occupancy for two years. In the meantime, she needed $25,000 as a down payment and some supplemental income to maintain her present home until her new place was completed. She had been feeling the pinch of not having her sister's income any longer to help pay for the upkeep of her house.

She took out a five and one-half year fixed-term RM with the intention of paying it off as soon as she was able to move into the retirement center. Under the terms of this loan, she received an initial disbursement of $33,000 to cover the down payment and closing costs for her new home at the retirement center, and to pay off a small lien on the home she already owns. She will receive $1,300 a month. The longer-than-needed term is a safeguard in case she is unable to move when she expects to move. There is no additional cost for taking the longer term, since when the loan is paid back she will only owe what has been disbursed plus the accumulated interest, whether she pays it back in one, two, or five years. There is some risk for Mrs. Valez since if her health should fail and she is no longer eligible for the retirement center, after five and a half years the lender would expect her to repay the loan. In this case, it is most likely that she would have to sell her house.[8]

A fixed-term RM is best suited for the person who needs additional monthly income for a limited and definite period of time and who intends or expects to sell the house when that time period is over.

As I said earlier, a variation of the fixed-term RM is a split-term RM, currently available only in two states, Connecticut and Rhode Island. This loan is called a split-term loan because the term of the loan advances is different from the term of the loan repayment. The monthly payments are guaranteed for a fixed number of years but are scheduled to stop at a specific time. However, when the term of payment ends the repayment of the loan does not start. In other words, until the homeowner dies or sells the house, repayment is not required. This is the main advantage over the fixed-term RM.[9]

A second major type of RM is called a "long-term or shared appreciation" loan, and is the only RM that provides monthly loan advances for as long as you live in your home and defers all repayment until you sell or die. In exchange for this open-ended income guarantee, the borrower agrees to pay the lender an amount of money equal to some or all of the future appreciation in the home's value. In this type of loan the factors affecting the size of the monthly advance to the homeowner include: the age of the borrowers, the status of the borrowers (i.e., single, married, or other joint borrowers), the value of the home, and the size of the appreciation share paid to the lender.[10]

Bernard Berg, an eighty-year-old widower, lived in a split-level house in a small town in the Midwest. The house had three bedrooms and one and a half baths. He had been an optometrist but was now retired. Mr. Berg had two children, a son and a daughter, and the thirty-three-year-old son was still living at home. The son has had some problems and is only marginally employable, so his father continues to support him. Bernard's wife died four years ago, about a year after he had retired. He has since put more time into community volunteering and recreational activities. He joined the local senior center and became quite a good amateur painter.

Life had settled into a pleasant routine. With his son at home, Bernard was not lonely. But two years ago, his son lost his job and has since been unable to hold any job, and then Bernard developed a chronic condition that requires frequent hospitalizations and expensive medical treatments. Because of these changes, Bernard depleted his savings and needed extra income in order to keep up with his large medical expenses and the support of his son. Very reluctantly, he decided that the only way to raise sufficient money to cover his needs would be to sell the house that he had lived in for his entire married life.

Bernard contacted a local real estate agent and shared his problems with her. She was most sympathetic and fortunately knew about a shared appreciation RM that was being offered by a national mortgage company. This RM would give him the extra monthly income he required and allow him to remain living in his own house for the rest of his life. His home was appraised at $300,000, and he gave the lending institution 100 percent appreciation. The interest rate was 14 percent. Bernard is receiving $1,000 a month and will continue getting this amount until he dies or sells the house, at which time the full amount of the loan plus the interest paid out will have to be repaid. However, no matter how large this repayment is, it cannot exceed 94 percent of the sale price less the appreciation. Mr. Berg is exceedingly pleased with this arrangement and is sorry that he had not known about the plan a few years ago since it would have made life a lot easier for him and his son.

Mrs. Mary Roth, a seventy-four-year-old widow, lived in a suburb of a small city in the East. Her small cottage was on a corner lot, and had a garage in the back. Her home consists of a work kitchen, dining room, living room, two bedrooms, and a bath. Mary's husband had owned a gas station. He became ill with a tumor on the spine in 1983. Despite an operation, he became completely paralyzed. He continued to live at home, with his wife taking care of him. In a short while, their savings and insurance were completely depleted and they were forced to borrow money in order to pay for his medical expenses. Since they had no children or other family who could help them out, they sank into debt. Mr. Roth died a few years ago.

The strain of taking care of a paralyzed spouse left Mary in poor physical shape. She became diabetic and needed a gall bladder operation. In addition, the house had been neglected during her husband's illness; the paint was peeling on the outside, the roof needed repairs, and both the plumbing and electrical systems needed to be fixed. She did not know what to do or where to turn for help but wanted to remain in the house she had called home for so many years. Fortunately, her plight had come to the attention of the local outreach worker (see chapter 6 for a discussion of the outreach program).

The outreach worker visited her at her home and quickly became aware of all her problems, including the fact that she needed money for oil to heat her house. He explained the various programs that she was eligible for and helped her apply for food stamps, home energy assistance, pharmaceutical assistance, etc. These programs, however, could not take care of the major repairs her home needed or her huge debt. The worker suggested that she should consider selling her house and moving into a nearby subsidized senior citizen project. He took her on a tour of one that had immediate openings. Mrs. Roth did not like this alternative because she found the rooms too small and the buildings too "institutional." But more importantly, she really wanted to remain in the home she had lived in for over fifty years.

Because Mary wanted to continue living in her own home, she was given information about the various HEC programs. Her outreach worker told her to think carefully before seeking a loan, but felt it was the best solution for her if she wanted to keep her home. Although she had a paid-up mortgage, no bank would give her a home equity loan because of her poor credit rating and her low income. Mary finally decided that she would apply for a shared appreciation RM loan. Her house was appraised for $48,500. Since she gave the mortgage company 100 percent appreciation, she was awarded $204 a month for as long as she remained in the house. However, since she needed a large sum of money to pay off her debts, she was also given a cash advance of $9,500. The loan was for seven years at 13.5 percent interest. Therefore, she had to pay back this loan at the rate of $198 a month. This left her with a net of $6.00 a month. Although her extra income is negligible, she is now debt-free and is able to manage on her Social Security and the benefits the outreach worker helped her to get. Mary is pleased with this arrangement and most happy to have a solution to remaining in her own home. In addition, after the $9,500 loan is paid off, her income will be increased to $204 a month.

Mrs. Jane Lawrence, an eighty-four-year-old widow, has lived in a modest house for over fifty years. Her husband died five years ago;

at that time (due to her frailty) a trust was set up with a bank as her guardian, to manage her affairs. Jane had no children or any other close relatives and depended entirely on the bank to take care of her finances. The bank hired a live-in housekeeper to cook, clean, shop, and generally oversee Mrs. Lawrence's personal care. In addition, they hired a man to do the gardening and other outside chores. Jane seemed to be managing quite well under this arrangement. She spent her days watching TV, doing the *New York Times* crossword puzzles, reading, and napping. However, after a few years of this expensive care, Mrs. Lawrence's trust fund was depleted. At this time, the bank felt that she should sell her house and move to a nursing home. Jane refused to do this and said: "I'm not leaving this home. I want to die here. This is where I have lived all my life."

Jane was physically frail but mentally very alert, so she decided to get legal help to fight her guardian's decision. She could not afford a private attorney, but she was fortunate to find a legal services agency in her community that had a "Friend Advocate Program." The program aide evaluated her personal care needs and determined that she was eligible for some community services that could take the place of her present expensive arrangement. The legal services agency arranged for her to receive "meals-on-wheels" five times a week, found a nursing student from a local college to do friendly visiting twice a week, secured a volunteer from a church to help with cleaning and laundry two days a week, and enlisted the aid of a Mr. Fixit program to take care of the outside chores (see chapter 6 for more information on these programs).

However, since Jane's income was so low and all her assets were gone, she needed additional monthly income to take care of some paid help and her other personal expenses. Because the bank had decided to put her in a nursing home and had the legal right to do this, and because the legal services agency believed that this decision was unwarranted, they decided to go to court to have the guardianship set aside so that Mrs. Lawrence could make her own decision about her living arrangement. The legal services agency won the case. Jane was overjoyed and felt that now she did not have to move to a nursing home. However, the problem of maintaining herself and her home on her insufficient funds still remained. The legal services lawyer researched Jane's problem and found an RM loan program that seemed to offer a good solution. The home was appraised for $82,000, and she gave 100 percent appreciation, since there were no relatives to whom to leave an estate. Since she was eighty-four years old, she was awarded $700 a month for the rest of her life, or until she sold her house. This amount was more than enough to provide for Jane's needs and she has continued to live in her own home.

-✠-

My final story concerning a shared appreciation RM is about Mrs. Dora Leipsig, a seventy-four-year-old widow. She lives in a suburban town in the South, where she has lived all her life. Indeed, she was born in a house two blocks away from where she now lives. She has lived in her present home for thirty-eight years. Her two-story house has a kitchen, living room, den-dining room, one bedroom, and a bath on the first floor, and two bedrooms on the second floor. It is attractively furnished and very well kept.

Dora is a sweet-looking, soft-spoken woman who speaks as if she has ill-fitting false teeth. She married at eighteen and raised two children. Her husband felt that women should not work but be at home. "My husband wanted me here when he left in the morning, and when he returned at night. But I really didn't mind since I enjoyed staying at home," she said. Dora did volunteer work as a nurse's aide at a local hospital for a number of years. Her husband worked as a foreman in a cement-block factory and apparently earned a good salary. She is close to her two sons; one lives just a few blocks away and the other lives in the next town, a ten-minute ride from her house. Her husband died almost twenty years ago and her children felt that she should sell the house and move in with one of them. But she decided not to rush into any move, but to wait a year before making any decision. On looking back, she feels she did the right thing, since she eventually decided to get rid of all her furniture and redecorated the entire house.

However, since she does not drive, and was lonely after her husband's death, she thought she should rent out a room or find someone compatible who also had a car to share the house with her. While she was mulling this idea over, she met Joe at a meeting, and he was looking for a new place to live. They seemed to hit it off and decided to try sharing Dora's house. They have since homeshared for seventeen years—needless to say, the sharing arrangement has worked out extremely well (house sharing will be discussed in the next chapter).

Mrs. Leipsig appears to be in relatively good health, but volunteered that eight years ago she had been very ill and required frequent hospitalizations. She was vague about the nature of her disease. She seems like a very active and social person and is friendly with most of her neighbors, who have lived in their homes for many years. When she is at home she enjoys gardening, sewing, TV, and some reading, although recently her eyes get very tired so that she has to limit reading. She enjoys her house and takes real pride in it, and recounted how she has recently repainted the interior walls downstairs.

Joe has turned out to be a real friend. He retired twenty years ago from a state civil service job and has been widowed for a long time. He has one son who lives near the shore, and he and Dora frequently visit this son and go out on his boat. Since Joe drives a car, they seem to be always going someplace, to the track, to the movies, and visiting friends and family. Aside from sharing the expenses of the house, Joe has been a big help because he does the outside work of mowing the lawn and shoveling the snow. Dora thinks that she is lucky to have found Joe, since so many of the widows she knows live alone and are always complaining about their neglectful children and how lonely they are. "Children have their own life to lead, with their families and their work, and they can't be at the beck and call of their parents. I'm very close to my sons and daughters-in-law and see them often, but I try not to ask them to be constantly doing things for me. In this way we really enjoy each other." She said this with a little smile and throughout our conversation displayed a delightful sense of humor.

Although Mrs. Leipsig receives Social Security, has a small amount of additional income from investments, and gets money from Joe for his share of the house expenses, she found that she needed a little more money to be able to continue her life-style. She said: "I have expensive tastes. I like going to the track, buying good perfumes, and giving costly gifts to my grandchildren. I also am a little worried about the fact that as I get older I may need more money for medical expenses." She began to look into home equity loans and when she discovered shared appreciation RM loans, she immediately applied for one. Her house was appraised at $95,000, and she gave 70 percent appreciation. For the past three years she has been receiving $200 every month. "I think this is wonderful," she said. "This money enables me to have the luxuries I couldn't have and also gives me something extra to put aside for illnesses." Dora also stated that both of her sons were well-off and they did not need an inheritance from her. At the end of the interview, Dora added that just two weeks ago she discovered that she needed a new roof, and would not have to put it off since she could now afford to have the roof fixed.

The last type of reverse mortgage I will discuss is called a line-of-credit RM. This loan does not give either a lump sum up front nor a constant monthly payment, but advances a line of credit for a maximum amount. Portions of this money can be withdrawn at any time but the number of payments per year are limited, and the amounts of these payments are also limited. Similar to the other kinds of RMs, this type does not have to be repaid until the owner dies or sells the house. The line-of-credit RM is advantageous to the elderly homeowner who has enough income to take care of his usual expenses but cannot meet any unexpected situations, such as a major house repair or a costly health problem. Unfortunately, only two states offer this program, Virginia and Maryland.[11]

The Virginia Housing Development Authority sponsors a senior home equity program that offers line-of-credit RM loans. They gave me the following examples to demonstrate how such loans are made. The first borrower was a 91-year-old widow who lived in a single-family detached dwelling. Her annual income was $5,146. Her house was appraised at $78,460. The maximum equity line was determined to be $50,000. The widow needed these funds to pay for medical expenses, taxes, and insurance.

The second borrower was an eighty-four-year-old single man who also lived in a single-family detached house. His annual income was $18,917. His house was assessed at $86,000. His maximum equity line was set at $34,400. He used this money to pay for in-home help. The third borrower was a married couple; the husband was seventy-six and his wife was seventy-five. They lived in a single family house, which was appraised at $28,900. Their yearly income of $15,189 was sufficient for their regular expenses, but they needed extra money to pay for some home repairs and improvements. Their maximum equity line was set at $9,537.[12]

To review briefly what I have been discussing in this chapter: In all the loan plans, the homeowner continues to own the house, and does not have to repay the loan plus the interest until the loan period ends or, in most cases, until he or she dies or sells the house.

Sale Leaseback

A second type of HEC plan I referred to at the beginning of this chapter is a form of sale called a sale leaseback. In a sale leaseback the homeowner sells his or her house to a buyer, with the understanding that he or she has the right to live in that house for as long as he or she wants to or until he or she dies. In other words, the homeowner now becomes a renter with a lifetime lease. The buyer becomes responsible for the maintenance, repairs, taxes, and insurance for the house, and pays the original homeowner a down payment and monthly payments for the duration of the loan. Although the new elderly renter now must pay rent to the buyer, in most cases, this rent is less than the monthly installment payments the renter receives as payments for the purchase of his or her house. Thus, until this loan is completely repaid, he or she has a net cash gain each month. The elderly seller also usually receives a substantial down payment which can be invested to give him or her additional income or he or she can buy a "deferred annuity" from a life insurance company. Payments from the annuity can be set up to start when the monthly payments from the buyer end.

Sale leaseback has never been as popular as the RMs because most of the elderly want to maintain their status as homeowners, and many older people find the idea of renting their own houses unappealing. In addition, the possibility of rent increases over the loan period tends to make older people uneasy. In the past few years interest by potential buyers willing to participate in this program has dropped because changes in tax law make it less profitable to own rental property.[13]

I did find one example of a sale leaseback. Mac, a man in his 50s, had a father who had a stroke and needed the kind of home care his mother could not provide. Since Mac's parents' home was their primary asset, and since they required a sizeable amount of money for an extended period of time to pay for his father's home care, Mac decided to purchase their home under a sale leaseback arrangement. The market value of his parents' home was $112,000. Mac paid $15,000 down and obtained a mortgage for the rest, then drew up a rental agreement with his parents. He made them a gift of the rent, however, so they paid nothing. Using the money gained from the sale of their house, Mac's parents bought a single-premium annuity that paid the elderly couple about $1,200 a month. They were also spared their former expenses of taxes, maintenance, and insurance, which Mac took over as new owner of the house. This extra income enabled his parents to hire the home health aides they needed. The costs, together with mortgage interest and depreciation, became tax deductions for Mac. In addition, he felt that the property was an excellent investment in a period of rising real estate values.[14]

Federally Insured Reverse Mortgages

Despite the apparent benefits of an HEC loan, only about 3,000 such loans have been made in the past ten years. Before that time, practically none were granted due to legal obstacles that have since been removed by federal legislation. But risks still remain for both lenders and elderly homeowners. Therefore, in 1987 Congress enacted a law creating a demonstration program that enables the Department of Housing and Urban Redevelopment (HUD) to insure up to 2,500 reverse mortgages (RM) to older homeowners by September 1991. It is expected that this law will help reduce the risks so that the number of HEC loans will increase dramatically.

The application process for these loans was begun in the fall of 1989. The new law states that "Elderly homeowners who are sixty-two years of age or older and who live in a home that they own free and clear (or almost free and clear) are eligible to apply for an FHA-insured reverse mortgage from a participating lender."[15]

These FHA-insured RMs allow the borrowers three basic payment options: "tenure, term, and line of credit." These options are the same as those already described in this chapter as long-term or shared appreciation, short-term, and line-of-credit. These insured RMs share similar features with the noninsured RMs, the elderly person remains the homeowner, and when the loan is due the lender cannot collect any more money than the sale price of the house. The big advantage of the insured loan is that the elderly homeowner "is protected if the lender fails to make the required payments under the mortgage."[16]

Another advantage is that in a shared appreciation loan, the monthly income to the homeowner should be higher because the reduced risk to the lender should result in a lower interest rate. A third advantage is that the borrower is not locked into a specific RM but can change to another type if changes in his or her life require a different financial arrangement. This type of flexibility, unique to the federal program, provides a very important advantage to the consumer. Another positive aspect of these RMs is that they will not be processed unless the older person has received counseling on the specific pros and cons of his or her particular situation. The AARP has trained several thousand volunteers and attorneys who can offer this type of counseling.

The main disadvantage of this federal demonstration program is that there is a cap on the income a borrower can receive. The maximum amount is $101,250, irrespective of the value of the house. Older people with homes that are worth more than $101,250, and who need higher loan payments than the maximum would allow, should find other alternatives.

Under this new program, the homeowner has to pay a mortgage insurance premium, so that the lender can recoup the loan in the event that the value of the house at the time of repayment is less than the amount of the mortgage loan. This is a two-part premium: the homeowner pays an initial 2 percent on the maximum claim amount, and then pays .05 percent of the mortgage balance each year.

The following is an example of how this insured program works:

Within the bounds of the principal limit, a borrower may select among alternative plans. For example, a seventy-five-year-old borrower in a $100,000 house with a 10 percent rate (and $3,500 in financed MIP and closing costs) could receive: a lump sum at closing of $41,600; tenure payments of $357 a month for as long as she or he lives in the house; term payments of $812 for 60 months; term payments of $510 for 120 months; or, combinations of the above. The risks to FHA and to the lender of all these options are the same, so the pattern of payments should be determined by the needs of the borrower. After consultation with the housing counselor and a lender, the borrower will be able to select the pattern best suited to his or her needs.

By statute, each potential borrower is required to discuss home equity conversion options and their alternatives with a HUD-approved counseling entity. HUD is using HUD-approved housing counseling agencies to provide counseling services for participants under the program. It is also certifying additional agencies that specialize in reverse mortgage counseling. HUD and the Administration on Aging have jointly funded training for counseling agencies to prepare them for their role in the demonstration.[17]

One of the first insured RMs issued was reported in an article in the *Times* (Trenton, N.J.) on November 5, 1989. It described a seventy-nine-year-old widow who had a modest income from Social Security and her husband's small pension. She and her husband had lived in their house for 15 years, and she had continued to live there since her husband died 19 years ago. The house has three bedrooms and the mortgage was paid off a year before she became a widow.

She was concerned about possible future medical expenses and wanted to be sure that she would not be forced to sell her home in order to pay for a long illness. This widow thoroughly enjoys her house, particularly working in her garden. She loves spending time with old friends, visiting, eating at restaurants occasionally, and going to the movies with them.

She plans to use the RM payments for nursing care in case of a protracted illness. "If you have cancer or something, it can really deplete savings, and then you become such a burden on other people," she said. "I just didn't want that."[18] However, initially, with the extra income she plans to fulfill a dream by taking a trip to Hawaii. She feels that having more cash to use while she is alive makes good sense; conversely, money obtained from the sale of her house after she dies would obviously not benefit her.[19]

Pros and Cons

I have now completed presenting the many different types of Home Equity Conversion (HEC) loans. My readers can see that if older people want to remain in their own homes but need a lump sum or additional monthly income, these loans are one way to meet their needs without having to sell the home. In addition, in most of these plans the elderly person continues to own the house and does not have to pay back the loan until the end of the loan period or until he or she moves or dies. The homeowner is never required to pay the lender more than the value of the house, even if the home's value shrinks over the years to the point that it is worth less than the original loan. More recently, the federal government has developed an insurance program that removes most of the risks associated with these loans.

Before you decide on any type of a home equity loan, you should ask yourself the following questions:

Do I want to continue to own my own home or would I be willing to sell it to someone else as long as I could remain in that home for the rest of my life?

Am I willing to forgo leaving the full value of my house in my estate for my children or other heirs?

Is my house costing me so much to maintain that I do not have enough money left for some necessities or pleasures?

Have I consulted my children and/or my lawyer about this plan?

Do I need a substantial amount of money for a major home repair?

Do I need long-term home health care that I can't afford?

Since all HEC loans use up some or all of the equity in the home, for those elderly who want to leave an estate for their children or other heirs, or who will need the money from the sale of their house for another living arrangement, HEC is not a viable alternative. Therefore, in the next chapter, I shall explore other programs that can offer the elderly increased income without sacrificing any of the equity in their homes.

3

No Longer Lonely

Accessory Apartments and Home Sharing

In the last chapter, I discussed how older people could exchange some of the equity in their houses for cash needed now without having to sell their homes and move. However, as I indicated, such complex arrangements may be objectionable to those homeowners who see them as mortgaging the future and diminishing their children's inheritance. Faced with income shortages, some may prefer renting out space in their homes, creating and renting an accessory apartment, or sharing the house with another person.[1]

The old adage, "There's nothing new under the sun," is only partly true. But the more you investigate modern living arrangements for the elderly, the more you will discover how few of the options are really new: many are just modern versions of past practices.

Anyone who lived through the Great Depression in a poor family will remember having to share a room with siblings in order to make room for a lodger or boarder. In those days, a space was often cleared to make room for a paying tenant who received a room and meals or kitchen privileges for his or her money. Often the tenant was an immigrant, a single person newly arrived in this country who needed inexpensive shelter until he or she could afford a place of his or her own. The lodger helped the hard-pressed family pay the rent or mortgage payment. No doubt this mutually beneficial, if somewhat inconvenient, arrangement continues among present immigrant populations. House sharing by singles and doubling up of families in areas where inexpensive housing is in short supply are the only ways some people can manage.

A more comfortable housing arrangement can be created, however, when homeowners are willing to share part or all of their houses or apartments with a tenant. A recent and helpful innovation is the "matching agency," a public or private agency that specializes in matching homeowners with home-seekers. By providing a central source of information and guidance, such agencies expedite the meeting of two segments of the elderly population with meshing needs: the homeowner in need of additional income, companionship, security, and possible services; and the home-seeker looking for affordable housing, security, and companionship. In addition, many house-matching agencies go beyond referrals and introductions, offering help to make these matches a success.

The shared space allotted to a renter may come in several forms: a room or two with bath and use of kitchen and living room in an apartment or house (home sharing), or a complete apartment in a house (accessory apartment).

Zoning restrictions in some towns and cities prohibit accessory apartments, but a growing movement demanding changes in these restrictive local laws may end this prohibition before too long. In those localities permitting such apartments, other factors have prevented proliferation, mainly (1) the desire for privacy, (2) a lack of knowledge and awareness by homeowners, and (3) the expense and inconvenience of conversion. Most often, it is serious financial need on the part of homeowners that pushes them to look for a tenant.[2]

The solutions of accessory apartments and home sharing not only provide the homeowner with additional income but can also supply companionship and help alleviate loneliness. In addition, the elderly renter who can not secure needed funds by means of a home equity loan can obtain needed cash from a home-sharing arrangement.

Adding an Accessory Apartment

Dorothy, the widow of a career naval officer, suffered a sudden drop in income after her husband's death. On the advice of a friend in real estate, she used her husband's life insurance money to pay for remodeling the upstairs bedrooms of her pretty saltbox cottage into a three-room apartment, keeping the five rooms on the first floor for herself and her precious collection of antiques. Dorothy found a tenant by contacting the county housing agency.

Since Dorothy valued her privacy, she was very fortunate to find a renter named Jenny, who had close family living near by. Because of this strong family relationship, Jenny did not need the friendship of her landlady. This suited Dorothy, who was mainly interested in earning income from the apartment. Her only concession to neighborliness was to knock on Jenny's door on mornings when she heard no sounds of movement upstairs. The two women exchanged sets of keys and emergency phone numbers and agreed to notify each other of overnight trips. Otherwise, they led completely separate lives, a situation entirely agreeable to both of them.[3]

Other housesharers and owners form closer relationships. Not long after Vera moved into the three-room apartment in the Green's house, the couple began to regard her as family. "Vera is like a sister to me," Rose said, describing how much she and her husband, Tony, liked Vera's company, how they regularly invited her to go shopping with them, and how she and Vera helped each other, exchanging recipes, knitting patterns, and soap-opera lore. Tony, a large, jovial man with a booming voice, agreed. "She's friendly and nice, and we all get along just great," he said.

All three were in their early seventies. Vera, widowed more than 30 years before, had no children. The Greens were the first family she had had in a long time. For Rose and Tony, having a tenant meant, in his words, "keeping the house that we love, our home for 32 years, the place where our son grew up." And the house—a neat red-brick split-level on a small manicured lot with trimmed yews and azaleas around the foundation and privet hedges on both sides separating it from neighboring lots—reflected their love.

Their only living child (one son had died in early childhood) lived a few blocks away with his wife and their three teenaged children. Rose and Tony were unusually doting grandparents, and the teenagers frequently stopped in, regarding the house as their second home. Rose and Tony's son, Greg, and his family had encouraged and helped with the conversion of the bedroom level into the apartment. Part of the first level was converted to a bedroom and bath for Rose and Tony, but the living room, dining room, and kitchen on the midlevel floor stayed the same. The house also had a partly finished basement.

"Plenty of room here. In fact, it's still too large for just two people. My Rose has a bum ticker and she shouldn't even be doing all the housework she does now," Tony said. He then proceeded to describe, with mock horror, the "mess and misery" they experienced during construction. "But I have no regrets," he hastened to assure me. "It was a good move. Not only can we keep the house, but we also have a little extra money for luxuries, like dinner out once in a while and travel." He mentioned two trips to his ancestral home in Italy and several weekend trips to scenic areas in the country with a local senior citizen's club.

Greg was more explicit about his parents' reasons for making the change. "My dad worked as a salesman for a big food company, and he retired with a pretty good pension and his Social Security. That was about seven years ago. But he soon discovered that his money didn't go very far, what with the price of everything, including taxes, going up. Then my mom had her heart attack, and that drained off more money. They were both really scared—about losing the house, about becoming a burden on me. So we came up with the idea for the apartment. And it's worked out real well. Now they feel secure about keeping the house, and they can also enjoy a few luxuries with the added income."

The house-matching agency contact was made by Greg, who wanted to be certain the renter would be a reputable person. "It may be a separate apartment, but it's still in the same house. And I wanted to be damn careful about who moved in," he said. He also realized, he explained, that if any serious problems developed, the agency could remove and relocate the tenant, something Rose and Tony would have great difficulty doing by themselves.

For both Vera and the older couple, this proved to be a mutually agreeable and profitable arrangement. Vera had a nice apartment at a reasonable rent, plus security and companionship. Rose and Tony gained greater security in their home and some discretionary income to improve the quality of their lives. As Tony said, "The best part is that our house still looks the same outside. And inside, it still feels like our house."[4]

Mrs. Janet Robbins, a widow for twelve years, is eighty-eight. She has two children, a son who lives close by and a daughter who is a nun and who can only visit infrequently. Her home is a lovely red-brick colonial that sits high on a hill set back off the road. The garden and plantings are beautiful, and the grounds are covered with wild laurel. The first floor has the usual living room, dining room, kitchen, and powder room; the second floor has three bedrooms and a bath. The couple built this house over fifty years ago and were very attached to it. Janet's husband was an electronic hobbyist and had a very large workshop.

After her husband died, Mrs. Robbins was lonely and concerned about her health. She wanted her privacy but also wanted someone in the house. So she decided to turn her husband's workroom into a studio apartment. It was large enough for a bedroom-living room, small kitchen, and a bathroom with a shower, but no tub. She found a very pleasant older woman to rent this apartment. Now she has a new friend, is no longer alone, and is earning needed income.

Sarah Gutmann is eighty-eight and has been a widow for fourteen years. She converted the second floor of her house into an apartment. Like the Greens, she and her renter have become so close that they go everywhere together. In addition the two of them are friendly with another pair of women who share a house (I will describe their situation following this story), and they have become a foursome for playing cards and taking trips.

Sarah was born in Europe, and was married there. She and her husband came to this country sixty-four years ago. She loves this country and said, "The minute I got off the boat I knew I would stay here—this is my country." Two years after the couple arrived in the United States, they brought over her parents and younger brother. Her parents lived with them until they died, and although she loved them dearly, she indicated that she would not want her children to be burdened with a similar situation. This seemed to be one of her reasons for creating an accessory apartment.

She has one married daughter who herself has five children and four grandchildren. So Sarah is a great-grandmother. Unfortunately, this family lives almost 1,000 miles away and therefore they can only see each other once or twice a year. When Sarah arrived in the United States, she could not speak English and had to take a job as a housecleaner. Her husband was a wood-carver and worked for himself. They settled in a city and he had a small workshop and made an adequate living. However, after a few years the rent became too high and they had to move. Her brother had settled in a rural part of the state and Sarah and her husband visited him frequently. They liked the area and decided to move there.

They built a two-story house with a living room, eat-in kitchen, two bedrooms, and a bath on the first floor, three small bedrooms and a bath on the second floor, and a large unfinished basement. They designed the upstairs to accommodate the family when they visit, and also felt it would be wise to rent one of the upstairs rooms for additional income. They had been fortunate to find teachers as boarders over the years.

After her husband died Sarah felt lonely and wanted someone living in the house who could be a real companion and also have a car, since she did not drive. Despite the fact that her brother lived just two houses away, Sarah did not want to become dependent on him since he had a wife and led a much different kind of life. But Sarah discussed her needs with her brother and he agreed that she should convert the upstairs into an apartment and look for a compatible tenant. Since her brother is a retired plumber, he was extremely helpful in deciding the least expensive way the apartment could be designed.

For the past thirteen years, Sarah has had Ruth, a seventy-two-year-old widow, as her tenant. The two women have become fast friends and go everywhere together. Ruth drives and has a car. Sarah is very involved in her church and actually met Ruth through her minister. The two of them have a very active schedule and spend most of their time away from home. Besides attending church regularly, they belong to its "ladies society" where they do needlepoint and raise money at flea markets and bake sales. They also do charity work and fund-raising for two religious organizations. Sarah is a past president of the ladies auxiliary of the American Legion and is now an honorary member. They attend all the dinners sponsored by the various local fraternal organizations.

In addition to their volunteer work, they do spend quite a bit of time on recreational activities. They attend the local senior citizen club's socials twice a month, and go on senior trips, such as the ballet at a performing arts center, and theater performances at the county community college. They also attend the local nutrition site for a midday meal on weekdays. Sarah said, "We don't go for the food. I go to help and be with people." She told me that she was a volunteer at the "meals program" run by the county when it first started 13 years ago, but that now she is just a participant. In addition to their activities, I got the feeling that they both were concerned about the plight of the other older people in their area and fought for their rights.

"I have lots of good friends," Sarah told me, and she and they spend some time visiting each other. Although Sarah and Ruth are out most days, they tend to be at home in the evenings. At night they do some light reading, watch TV together, and play cards or Scrabble. They get their exercise regularly since they take long walks each evening after dinner. "In the daytime, we have no time," Sarah offered with a smile.

Sarah is delighted with her present living arrangement and feels that she was really lucky to find a friend like Ruth. It was apparent that she was enjoying life and seemed quite spry for her age. She displayed a good sense of humor and made many sly comments. It is obvious that adding the upstairs apartment has not only given Sarah extra income, but it has provided her with a good friend who has enriched her life.

"So long as I can afford it, I won't move. I'm so glad that I don't need my children," she told me as I was leaving.

Not only did I have the good fortune to interview Sarah Gutmann and learn how her accessory apartment had enabled her to remain in her own home, but I unexpectedly had the opportunity to meet two of her closest friends. These people, Frances and Blanche, were living together in the same house, but from the onset had designed a two-family house.

Frances and Blanche were first cousins and had grown up together in the same neighborhood. There were good friends as well as family members. When the two women married, they and their husbands became a close foursome. So much so, that when Blanche was widowed fairly early in life, she continued to be very close to Frances and her husband and they visited frequently and went out together very often.

A few years after her husband died, Frances and Blanche and her husband decided to buy a vacation home in a rural area and convert it into a two-family house. They bought it jointly since they both wanted it to be their permanent home after retirement. Four years later, Frances's husband took early retirement and they moved into their vacation home. Blanche continued to use the house on weekends and vacations and she, too, moved in permanently on her retirement.

The house consists of two complete living units, one on each floor. Frances lives on the first floor and has a living room, dining room, large eat-in kitchen, bedroom, bath, and a "junk room." Blanche's apartment is on the second floor and has a living room, dining room, small eat-in kitchen, bedroom, and bath. Although there are two separate outside entrances, one gets the impression that since the death of Frances's husband, they tend to use the entire place as one living unit.

Frances and Blanche carefully planned their present living arrangement many years ago, since they wanted to be sure to have companionship and mutual support in their later years. Since they are now both in their late seventies and widowed, they seem very pleased with their present situation, have remained close, and spend most of their waking hours together. They usually eat breakfast in their own apartments, attend the nutrition site where they visit with their friends, particularly Sarah and Ruth, and use a large lunch as the main meal. In the evening they eat a light supper together in Frances's apartment. In fact they tend to spend most evenings together in her unit. Frances knits and crochets, while Blanche hooks rugs. Blanche added, "I like to do things fast. I don't have much patience for knitting or crocheting." Frances countered with, "She's a hooker," and they both laughed at her comment.

Blanche confessed that she really enjoys housecleaning which Frances finds strange. But Blanche said, "I don't do windows," and again they both chuckled at this remark.

It is obvious that they enjoy each other's company but also enjoy meeting and visiting with other people. When the lunch was over, Frances, Blanche, Sarah, and Ruth had a date to spend the rest of the afternoon together. They do this several times a week and look forward to this regular activity. Today, they were going to Frances and Blanche's house to play pinochle. They play for money and put the winnings in a pot. When they have accumulated enough cash, they go to a restaurant for dinner. These four women have only modest incomes, but they have found a way to enjoy life with limited money. Their mutual friendship and activities have enriched their lives, which have been reinforced by their housing arrangements.

-✳-

My last story about an accessory apartment concerns a widow in her late seventies who, unlike the other women I have met, had a different reason for adding on an apartment to her home. Her name is Lillian Ryan and she, her husband, and younger daughter moved to her present home twenty-five years ago. It is a hillside ranch on an acre lot, located in a very lovely university town. When they moved into this house her daughter was still attending high school. Their older daughter had just married and was living in a neighboring state.

Lillian's husband had been a successful businessman so that although she had worked as a social worker before her marriage, there was no economic reason for her to continue working outside the home. She stayed home and raised her two daughters, but became active in various community organizations, such as the Girl Scouts, the church, and PTA. The family also took extensive and frequent vacations and traveled throughout the United States.

Her husband died sixteen years ago while her younger daughter was away at college. This daughter continued to live away from home after she graduated. Since the daughter did not want to live with her mother, Lillian felt that she might move back home if she was offered a separate apartment. Lillian had been very close to her children, and now with her husband gone she really missed them.

Lillian's house was all on one floor. The main part of the home consisted of a living room with an L-shaped dining area, eat-in kitchen, three bedrooms and two baths, small den, and an attached two-car garage. It was important for Lillian to keep the main part of her house intact, so she decided that she could do without the garage and the den, a room her husband had used as his office. She had these two spaces converted into an attractive three-room apartment.

Although she now had a separate living unit to return home to, Lillian's daughter decided to stay in the other state where she had made many friends and found a good job. Since Lillian did not need the income from this apartment, she left it empty in the hope that her daughter would change her mind. After five years, the situation remained unchanged. Meanwhile Lillian was being pressured by friends to rent the apartment since apartments were in great demand in the community.

Lillian first rented the unit to a female graduate student, but when this tenant left, she realized that it would be helpful to have someone available for snow shoveling, putting out the garbage, and doing some heavy gardening chores. She found a young couple who were most anxious to rent and did not have much money; they readily agreed to pay a reduced rent in exchange for doing needed chores. She has had several tenants in the past eight years, since she lives in a very mobile community, but they have all been required to help with outside tasks.

This arrangement has not only provided Lillian with some important maintenance services at no cost, but it has also allowed her to take some deductions from her income taxes. This has saved her money because she has a sizable income. "The apartment is considered one-third of my house and therefore I can deduct one-third of my costs for heating, utilities, and repairs of the entire house. Also, I can deduct 100 percent of the repairs and maintenance of the apartment, and yearly depreciation of the cost of the conversion. In this way, I consider that all these deductions pay for my real estate taxes."

Lillian has a car and still drives. She says, "Mobility is most important in a suburban town, and I must be able to continue to drive in order to do all the things that I like to do. This being able to get around contributes to my independence of action and I don't have to put pressure on my friends for favors."

She is still an active participant in the community, and does volunteer work for the local historical society, the library, and the senior center, and is on the board of directors of two national women's organizations. In addition, she plays bridge at least twice a week and attends luncheons, dinners, and receptions sponsored by local churches and other community groups. She has continued to be an avid traveler, takes trips to Europe at least once a year, and spends six weeks in California or Florida each winter.

Lillian thoroughly enjoys her home. She says, "It gives me active pleasure. It represents my changing interests and my growth in the past 20 years. My house is very meaningful to me. I need all this space to accommodate my husband's and my children's things which are stored in my large basement. These are important links to my family for me. Also, I love my garden and am still able with my tenant's help to do some planting. Moving would represent a compromise which I'm not prepared to make. As long as I'm able to get around, I don't see any advantages to other housing arrangements."

Lillian is pleased with the financial benefits of her accessory apartment. She also has a stronger sense of security because she knows that her tenant(s) is close at hand if she needs help. Although she has been in relatively good health, she has had a few problems over the past two years that required her to use some homemaking services. Lillian did not find these particularly satisfactory. She is already thinking ahead and wondering if she should plan to use the apartment in a different way. "Perhaps I ought to think about what I would do if I can't manage like I'm doing now and will need help in maintaining my independence. Maybe I should open up the common wall between the house and the accessory unit and rent it to a couple. They could use it rent-free or at a greatly reduced rent, and in exchange the man would do all the outside work and his wife would do the cooking, shopping, and cleaning, as needed, and if or when I'm bedbound, they would take care of me."

If you are considering creating an accessory apartment, you should ask yourself the following questions:

Is my house designed so that I can easily and relatively inexpensively convert part of it into a separate apartment?

Can there be a separate private entrance for the new unit?

Would it bother me to have my house divided into two units?

Will I be left with enough living space to accommodate my own and my family's needs?

Do local zoning laws permit a second unit in my area? If not, do I have the patience to go through a variance procedure?

Is it important for me to have someone living in my own building whom I can call in case of an emergency and still maintain my privacy?

Will I mind the mess and clatter while the renovation takes place?

Home Sharing

Accessory apartments have been very good solutions for all the people I have described and have enabled them to continue living at home by providing them with extra income and, in some cases, companionship and support. However, there is another major alternative arrangement, called "home sharing," that can also supply these supports and additional money without making structural changes in the home. As I said earlier, a generation or so ago home sharing was known as "taking in a boarder." In a home-sharing arrangement, the homeowner reserves a private room and bath for his or her own use, gives the tenant a private room and bath, and shares the rest of the house. Usually, the tenant pays half the cost of maintaining the home as his rental fee.

Martha, age seventy, has never worked, had always been completely dependent upon her husband (a car dealer), and had enjoyed a life of luxury. Her only child, a son, had died in an auto accident when he was forty. His only son, Martha's grandson, lived in the southern part of the country; he telephoned and visited only rarely. Her husband's family and her friends were attentive but could not rid her of the depression and confusion that followed her husband's death the year before. The house seemed cavernous; as she said, "I feel like a small pebble in a huge, empty drum." When her husband's niece, who lived nearby and worked for a local family service agency, took her to see the director of the home-share program, she was ready for a housemate. Meanwhile, another widow, Charlotte, had already visited the agency with her daughter and left an application.

Charlotte had very little money to spend on rent. But Martha did not need money. She was offering two rooms (sitting room and bedroom with bath) plus the run of the living areas rent-free. In addition, she would pay $100 per month in exchange for services. What Martha hoped for was an efficient house manager to cook, shop, and organize the household. And that's what she found in Charlotte.

Relieved of most household responsibilities, Martha was generous in her praise of Charlotte's competence and good nature. "I'm not very good company these days," she admitted, "but Charlotte is always patient and tries hard to cheer me."

Charlotte said that Martha was often despondent, "though not as often as when I first came to live here. It takes some longer than others to come to terms with the loss of a husband. And when she gets a really bad crying jag, I call her niece or the social worker at the home-share agency."

The social worker called monthly to check on the progress of the pair and to discuss any problems. She seemed to think they were doing very well, although in her professional opinion, which she had conveyed earlier to Martha and her niece, Martha would have done better to sell her house and move to a congregate or life-care community or to a residential hotel. Martha could well afford one of these options but was adamantly opposed to giving up her house.

She and Charlotte were from different socioeconomic backgrounds. Their relationship was more like servant and mistress than one of peer companions. The binding factors in their relationship were almost entirely practical. Martha relied on Charlotte to run her household and to be a dependable presence in case of emergency. Charlotte received free room and board and an additional sum every month, all of which were a welcome supplement to her small government pension, enabling her to establish gift funds for her grandchildren, help her daughter with some of the family's disastrous finances, and buy a few extras for herself. She was very pleased with the way things worked out. "My only big wish right now," she concluded, "is for Martha. May the good Lord give her a happier heart."[5]

—❈—

Where difficult personalities are involved in a home-sharing match, the role of an agency is even more critical. Such was the case of eighty-five-year-old Inez, who came to live with sixty-eight-year-old Lucy.

Inez had lived in an apartment with her daughter and son-in-law for twenty-two years, but then her daughter developed terminal cancer. When her son-in-law gave up the apartment to move in with his own daughter, Inez hoped to be taken in by one of her other four grandchildren. Upset by their mother's illness and resentful over what they regarded as her years of sacrifice to Grandmother Inez, none of the grandchildren was willing to have her. They tried but were unable to find an apartment for her in a senior citizens' housing project. An appeal to the regional social services agency led to a referral to the county housing department's home-matching service.

Realizing that Inez was a dependent person and an unwilling participant in the arrangement, the service tried to choose a younger, more stable homeowner as a partner. This was not an easy task: older homeowners often prefer younger renters, but younger homeowners rarely request older tenants.

Lucy, a recently retired high school math teacher, had lived in her house for almost forty years, ten of them as the widow of a college sociology professor. After her retirement, she found taxes and maintenance of the house too costly and applied to the agency for a tenant who could have her own bedroom and bath and share the rest of the house. Thus began a rocky relationship.

To begin with, Lucy complained that Inez expected to be waited on. "She wants me to do all the shopping and cooking, to serve the meals and clean up afterward, too. Then she's always asking me to drive her here and there. I didn't ask for a tenant in order to become a housemaid and a chauffeur."

Inez appealed for sympathy: "I'm old and sick. I have no strength. I still haven't gotten over this move. I'm ready to have a nervous breakdown. But you won't have to put up with me much longer. My grandchildren are coming for me soon."

With the agency's intervention, Lucy and Inez came to an agreement that was put into writing. Each would shop and cook separately; Inez would be responsible for cleaning her own room, bath, and the kitchen when she used it; Lucy would be responsible for the rest of the house; and Inez would pay Lucy a small sum for transportation.

Three years later, the two were still together, still squabbling over petty annoyances:

"Lucy, your cats are on my bed again."
"Inez, I've told you a hundred times to shut your door if you don't want them there."
"Lucy, you left dirty dishes in the sink again last night."
"I was too tired to do them."
"Too drunk you mean."

And so it went. But like an old married couple, they seemed to have settled into a state of contentious equilibrium—and even to have grown fond of each other.

Would this home-share arrangement have survived the earlier disagreements without the agency's mediation and written contract? It is difficult to say. Lucy, the homeowner, might easily have turned Inez back to the agency, creating untold hardships for Inez and her family.

The grandchildren were pleased with the arrangement, despite all Inez's earlier complaints. "Grandma's a much nicer person now," one granddaughter claimed. "Being with Lucy has made her stand up for herself, instead of depending on my parents all the time, the way she used to. She and Lucy are more like equals. And talking with the agency counselors has probably helped her a lot, too."

This granddaughter and another who lived nearby stopped in occasionally for coffee and a chat, sometimes bringing one or two of their children. At least one of them took Inez shopping once each week and made certain she was driven to all family gatherings and festivities. Lucy, who had no children of her own, enjoyed the family visits almost as much as Inez did and was sometimes invited to family gatherings.[6]

-✵-

Mrs. May Bland found her roommate through Operation Match in Rockville, Maryland. She owned a townhouse and worked part-time as a real estate agent. Unfortunately, she was in a bad financial situation due to inflation and a slow real estate market that had led to a drop in her income. The match agency was able to find her another older woman to share the house and all the expenses with her. She says, "This is working out beautifully. I don't know how I would have been able to keep my townhouse without having Joan as my house sharer." She was pleased at being able to maintain her home and to have found a new friend.

Operation Match does not charge fees. Mrs. Bland explained how the service worked. "First they interview you and ask many questions about your home, how you want to share, and what kind of financial arrangement you want. In addition, they ask you your personal preferences about drinking, smoking, and the like." After the interview Mrs. Bland received a questionnaire. Two weeks later, she was given the names and phone numbers of five older women the agency thought would make suitable sharees for May. The first person she called was Joan and she seemed to be the right age and had similar interests. May invited her to see the house and meet with her. After this visit they mutually agreed to try a home-sharing arrangement which has been working out extremely well.[7]

Mrs. Warrington's husband died two years ago, when she was seventy. She has two sons who are both married and have children of their own. On her limited Social Security income she found it difficult to maintain her home. Also, being alone, especially at night, proved to be frightening. Mrs. Manley, a sixty-eight-year-old widow, could not afford to pay a large rent increase and was looking for a less expensive living arrangement. Sharing Mrs. Warrington's three-bedroom house seemed like a good solution. They take their meals together and share the household tasks. Indeed, the arrangement seems to be working perfectly:

> They exchange favorite recipes. . . . Mrs. Warrington says, "You can't measure all the home-sharing benefits in dollars and cents. . . . It's worth an awful lot to get a good night's sleep because there's another person in the house."
>
> Mrs. Manley adds, "I'm so happy that I found a companion and good friend as well as a comfortable place to live."[8]

In addition to peer home sharers, there are intergenerational arrangements. These usually involve both companionship and services in exchange for little or no rent. Mrs. Peterson, age eighty-two, had a serious heart condition. She refused to go to a nursing home since she wanted to remain in her home. Her friends and family were worried about her living alone and convinced her to find someone to share her house who could help her with the heavy work that she was not able to do anymore.

Mrs. Peterson agreed, and with the help of a home-match agency she found a graduate student named Steven. The student could only afford a cheap rent and needed a quiet place to study. Now he gets his housing rent-free; in exchange he does all the gardening and cleans the house.

> Mrs. Peterson remarks, "What a joy to have a young person around. It's not just the help but the lovely sounds of life in my house once again."
>
> Steven says, "Mrs. Peterson is a real survivor; I admire her a lot. She has given me the opportunity to continue my studies even though tuition has doubled in one year."[9]

A successful match sponsored by a Seattle agency involved a seventy-nine-year-old widow named Hattie DuRuz and a young man in his late twenties named James Giga. He had just started his practice as a chiropractor and after paying for his office equipment needed a low rent in order to stay in business. Hattie provided a comfortable place for him to live at a nominal rent of $150 a month. He feels as if Hattie is a substitute grandmother and enjoys this relationship, while Hattie feels that James supplies the security and company that she needs in addition to his rent which helps with her bills.[10]

Another unusual intergenerational match involves a young graduate student, Joe Fine, and a seventy-five-year-old widow, Lois Baer. Lois was recovering from a hip operation and she was finding it extremely hard to perform her household chores. She did not want to move to an adult home because she wanted to remain independent and in control of her own life. A friend told her about Philadelphia Match, which connects homeowners with younger people looking for a place to live.

Joe not only found the family-oriented living arrangement that he had been looking for, but since he was studying social work, he has gained a new understanding of what it means to be old. Lois feels that without Joe she could not have remained in her house or else she would have become overly dependent on her family and friends. Neither of these situations would have been acceptable to her.

As the year progressed, their relationship deepened. At first, it was more like a grandmother-grandson relationship, but then they established a real mutual support system and friendship. Lois even confessed that although Joe is so much younger she continues to learn about new things from him. And, of course, Joe feels that Lois, with all her experience, is a tremendous help in solving his problems.

Lois did confess that, at first, she was not too sure that sharing her house with a person fifty years younger than herself would really work. She was looking for a nonsmoker who would not balk at housecleaning, grocery shopping, and emptying the cat litter tray. She also wanted someone with a car who would be available to take her out each day. Since no available older person could fill the bill, she reluctantly accepted Joe as a housemate. She is now thoroughly convinced that she made the right choice and feels that society ought to provide more opportunities for the old and the young to mix. When Joe graduates and moves to another town she will miss him, but plans to ask for a similar student to replace him.[11]

Although it is more usual to pair people of similar ages in a house-share arrangement, some agencies will make intergenerational matches. Indeed, a few agencies even specialize in this service. One such agency, SHARE (Student Housing Alternative with Rural Elders), is located in California, Pennsylvania. Its mission is to pair students and older homeowners in shared housing. The program has been most successful, producing all the benefits that have been described above.

Although the first home-sharing agency was established in Hartford, Connecticut, in 1953, it was not until the mid- to late 1970s that this type of housing arrangement began to flourish. Another agency, also called SHARE (Senior Housing At Reduced Expense), became operational in 1977. This is run by the Family Service Association of Nassau County, New York, and became the model for many other match agencies in the country. It feels that the key to a successful home-sharing arrangement is the careful matching of the two people involved.

SHARE operates as follows:

When a homeowner first applies for a house-sharer, he or she comes to the office and is interviewed. A detailed description of the homeowner's preferences in terms of interests—smoking, drinking, other habits, hobbies, disabilities, and special needs—is recorded. Similar information is collected from those people wanting to share a home. This information is placed on file cards, with one set of cards filed alphabetically, and another according to house location. The cards are color-coded by homeowner and by tenant.

Following the interview, a staff member makes a home visit and records a complete description of the house. This includes size and number of rooms, available closet space, linens, kitchen equipment, storage space, and general condition of the house. The staff then selects an appropriate match and the two clients are informed. If they are interested in pursuing an arrangement, they are given each other's phone numbers and do the rest themselves.

Follow-up phone calls are made by the agency a few weeks after the tenant moves in, and again a month later. Although there may be informal contacts later on, the agency usually does not interfere unless the homeowner or sharer asks for assistance.

There is no fee for this service and the agency is careful not to influence either party in the home-share process. The sharers are the sole decision makers in determining whether they want a share arrangement and whether they will be compatible. On the whole the agency finds that often a homeowner who initially asked for a house-sharer, when faced with the real situation, may become somewhat apprehensive. Counseling is often helpful in these situations. Sometimes the prospective tenant also needs counseling to deal with moving into someone else's home. It has been the agency's experience that careful selection and initial counseling usually make for successful matches.[12]

A recent study of home sharing indicates that the most important reasons given for choosing this type of living arrangement are finances, need for services, and companionship.[13] The role of the matching agency was found to be critical in the success of these matches, since the agency can provide case management services and can help resolve any conflicts between homeowners and home-sharers. In addition, it can arrange for new matches so that the homeowner can continue to remain at home even if he or she requires a succession of home-sharers. The study concluded that home sharing was a beneficial alternative for the elderly in need of extra income, or support services, or companionship. In addition, they found that this type of arrangement reduced the strain on the caregiving family members.

The Shared Housing Resource Center has suggested some specific questions for those older people who are considering sharing their homes or apartments. The following is their self-questionnaire:

Why do I want to homeshare with someone?

Is my home or apartment suitable for sharing? For example, is there a private room for a housemate? Is there an easily accessible bathroom? Is there adequate closet or storage space? Are there structural barriers, such as stairs, that might limit who can live in my home?

Is the space I'm making available ready for another person(s) and their possessions? If not, what must I do to make it ready? Will the space be furnished or unfurnished?

If a person needs an unfurnished bedroom, am I willing to store my things?

How much rent do I need in order to satisfactorily reduce my housing cost burdens?

Would I need some help around the house? If yes, how much assistance do I need?

If I expect a service, should I reduce the rent, offer free rent, free room and board, or free room and board plus compensation for the services a housemate would provide?

Am I prepared to adjust to some household changes in return for the additional income or help that I am asking?

To what degree do I want to share my kitchen, living room, and other common areas?

What household responsibilities do I wish to share? For example: housework, cooking, shopping, driving, gardening, trash removal, handiwork, laundry, etc.?

What are my housekeeping standards? For example, how clean should common areas be kept?

Am I willing to provide any services? For example: cooking, laundry, driving, etc.?

What is essential to me in a housemate:
  Do I prefer a female, male, couple?
  Do I have an age preference?
  Would I consider living with children?
  Do I have a racial or religious preference?
  Do I object to smoking or drinking?
  Would I consider living with pets?

What kind of relationship do I want with my housemate? Do I just want a tenant/landlord relationship, or do I want a friendly companion with whom to share my life?

Do I have specific interests I would like to share with my housemate?

What are my shortcomings that might present difficulties to anyone living with me?

What qualities do I have that would contribute to a shared arrangement?

What can I do to ensure that *my* home can become *our* home when shared with another?[14]

In summary, it is advisable that a person who is considering home sharing should clarify his or her expectations and make sure that he or she gets to know the potential sharee well enough so that the two of them can live together. In addition, the two people need to feel that they are each gaining from this living arrangement and that it is mutually satisfactory.

Shared Housing Cooperatives

A third possible alternative that combines some of the features of the accessory apartment and home sharing is called a shared housing cooperative. I have found no examples of such an arrangement, but it could be created by a homeowner who is looking for additional income and a family-style living arrangement.

If an older homeowner has a very large house, that is, one that has at least four bedrooms and two baths, it can be converted into two or three studio apartment units or into two to four bedroom and bath suites. These can be rented, or the owner can decide to offer cooperative ownership shares to the other occupants. Of course, in the latter case, the original homeowner is no longer the sole owner but owns a share in the house, along with the other occupants.

This arrangement would have the distinct advantages to the original homeowner of realizing a substantial amount of cash from the sale of the shares, increasing the number of owners to share in maintenance and repair costs, and adding several people for support and companionship. On the other hand, in a cooperative ownership arrangement, the original homeowner would need to consult with a knowledgeable lawyer and perhaps seek the help of a local non-profit agency with experience in group-shared residences or home sharing. The latter is important since, unless the homeowner shares the house with friends or people he or she has known, this can be difficult to work out with total strangers.

There are models of shared cooperative living arrangements in the communal housing that students and other young people have developed. Many of these have worked quite well and have existed for long periods of time.

Financing Accessory Apartments

Accessory apartments require financing or a cash outlay for the necessary renovation, while home sharing does not usually require capital outlays for structural changes to the house. There are various methods of raising money to cover the costs of creating an accessory apartment, which can run from $15,000 to $25,000, depending on the area of the country in which the house is located and the amount and type of renovations required. The most obvious way to raise the necessary cash is to take out a home equity loan from a bank. The monthly payments can be made from the rent received from the apartment. As described in the previous chapter, a reverse mortgage deferred payment loan or line-of-credit loan can also raise the cash needed for renovation. In addition, many state finance agencies and local community housing agencies have programs that lend money for house renovations at low interest rates. In some cases the borrower's income has to fall within a specified range.

A new lending program has just been announced by the federal government. It is administered by Fannie Mae with an allocation of "$100 million to fund mortgages through Seniors' Housing opportunities." Now only a demonstration project, it hopefully will become an on-going program. Accessory apartments and home sharing are among the eligible housing alternatives that can be funded. The specific requirements and a list of lenders can be obtained from Fannie Mae (see appendices).

Generally, the homeowner must be at least 62 years old, and must demonstrate the ability to pay off the loan. However, the anticipated rental income from the prospective tenant could be used to qualify for the mortgage. "To finance an accessory apartment, the occupant of the principal unit must be a senior or a relative of a senior."[15]

Pros and Cons

Both accessory apartments and home sharing have been good solutions for some elderly who want to remain in their own homes. As I have indicated, these people have derived the benefits of added income and social support and security. However, there are some disadvantages to these arrangements that must be carefully evaluated before making a decision.

Some older people do not feel that the added income is sufficient to compensate for the loss of part of their house or the inconvenience during the period of renovation. Some do not really believe that after paying the increased taxes, insurance, and maintenance costs there will be any rent gain from the rent. And others do not want any other person living in their house, even in a separate apartment. Some of the elderly fear making any change in their living arrangement, and are skeptical about doing anything that has not been proven over a long period of time. Some elderly people feel that creating an apartment in their home might lower the property's value, and eventually reduce their children's inheritance. In addition, some adult children disapprove of their parents making any major changes to the family home.

In the case of home sharing, the obvious disadvantages are the lack of privacy and the sharing of one's home with a stranger. However, if the need for additional income or for added security and companionship is compelling, then these disadvantages become unimportant.

On the whole, I found that both accessory apartments and home sharing provided excellent solutions and have helped many older people remain in their own homes.

4

Sprucing Up the Homestead
Home Maintenance and Repairs

Not only are financial assistance, social support, and companionship important in enabling older people to remain in their own homes but the house must be maintained and kept in good repair so that it continues to be a suitable place to live. Therefore, the elderly need assistance obtaining appropriate workmen and, in some cases, financial help to pay for maintenance and repair services.

Many small businesses in the repair industry are marginal operations, in business today, bankrupt tomorrow. Elderly homeowners are often "ripped off" by workmen who do a poor job, start a job but never finish it, or overcharge for the work done. Sometimes the work need not have been done in the first place. Door-to-door solicitors are experts at preying on the fears of the elderly and know how to use scare tactics such as, "Your foundation is collapsing—if it is not repaired immediately, your house will fall down."

It may be difficult for an elderly person who finds himself victimized by an unscrupulous repair service to get help from a family member because he or she may be unaware of the situation. The parent may be reluctant to tell his children about problems with repair and maintenance people for fear that they will think he or she is becoming incompetent and is no longer able to manage at home. To avoid dealing with dishonest contractors, the elderly should contact the appropriate local housing agency to obtain a list of reputable repair services in their area. Some agencies also offer follow-up services to ensure that the homeowner is not exploited.

Keeping one's home in a good state of repair is important at any stage of life, but particularly important as one gets older. The elderly spend much more time at home and are more accident-prone because they experience losses in vision, hearing, touch, smell, muscular coordination, physical strength, and mobility due to the aging process and chronic illness.

Ann, a widow in her early eighties, almost waited too long to do the necessary repairs on her house. If not for the intervention of her daughter, Marlene, the house would have deteriorated to such an extent that Ann would have been forced to give up her home. Marlene and her mother had not had a good relationship since her childhood, because she felt that she was "nagged all the time to be tidy" and continually reminded of her failings. She was very attached to her father, who died at an early age. Thereafter the bad feelings between mother and daughter grew worse. Despite this hostility between Marlene and Ann, when Marlene became aware of the bad condition of her mother's home she knew that something had to be done.

Inside, Ann's home was the neat, pretty little house she had lived in for almost sixty years. Outside, however, the walls appeared to be tumbling down. Boards were rotting, and the front porch and steps sagged dangerously. Some of the storm windows had been removed; others were broken or warped and thick with years of accumulated grime.

Since Marlene was unable to get her mother to do anything about fixing the house she decided to seek help with a local family service agency. At first, Ann refused to allow the agency worker into her house, but after several phone calls she reluctantly agreed to admit her. Inside, every article was clean and meticulously placed. Ann proudly proclaimed that she spent most of her waking hours dusting, washing, and polishing the downstairs rooms, where she lived. (The two upstairs bedrooms were closed off.) But even the interior was sorely in need of paint and repairs: faucets dripped, ceiling and wall plaster was flaked and crumbling, linoleum was cracked, and rugs were threadbare.

Ann herself, a tall bony woman, seemed weak and emaciated. Her steel-gray hair was pulled back tightly and coiled into a bun; her dress was neat, but spotted and mended; her shoes were worn at the toes and at the heels. She angrily asked whether Marlene had "foisted" the agency on her and insisted she could "manage quite well without any help, thank you."

After several visits, the agency worker was able to allay some of

Ann's suspicions. By appealing to her sense of pride in her home, she convinced the older woman to apply to a nonprofit neighborhood housing committee that offered maintenance and repair services. Services provided for elderly, handicapped, and low-income homeowners included carpentry, plumbing, masonry work, winterization, roofing repairs, and window replacement. Most of the work was done free of charge or for a small fee, with funding from various sources, such as United Way, community development block grants, state funds, and foundation grants.

Because of a long list of applicants, it would be at least six months before work was started on Ann's house. And so far, she had given her approval only for exterior repairs. If Marlene wished, the caseworker would try to persuade Ann to accept interior work as well.

The family service agency also arranged for Ann's house to be registered with the neighborhood crime-watch group; it was now on the regular patrol route. Ann had been listed with a church reassurance service that would telephone daily as a safety check.

Best of all, the caseworker had established enough trust with Ann to take her shopping twice a week. The first thing they did was to buy Ann a new pair of shoes.

Marlene believed that her mother feared going out alone in her crime-ridden neighborhood and consequently curtailed her shopping until she reached the point of starvation. Marlene brought her groceries periodically, but face-to-face encounters were so unpleasant that she visited her mother as infrequently as possible. She was happy to pay the agency worker for her time as a shopping companion and to confine her own filial duties to weekly phone calls. "What a load off my mind!" Marlene said. "It's almost as if I'd found a long-lost sister to take over the care and coddling of mother."[1]

-⁂-

Another elderly woman I met at a nutrition site did not have any family who could intercede on her behalf, and her home was also in need of extensive repairs. She told me that while she held a job she was able to keep up with the necessary repairs. But since her retirement she had not been able to do this and so her house was rapidly deteriorating. She refused to apply for any local funds since she equated this with "welfare."

Her house needed insulation. The windows needed caulking, especially in the upstairs rooms. In the cold weather—which in up-state New York where she lives can last five or six months—her pipes freeze because she turns off her heat upstairs in order to save money on her utility bills. She closes the upstairs and sleeps down-stairs on a makeshift bed in the living room.

I spoke to the nutrition site director who told me that she had been trying to talk this woman into applying for funds that were available to repair the windows and add extra insulation. In addi-tion, she was eligible to receive help with her heating bills. So far, the staff has not been successful because the older woman has a fierce pride and refuses to accept any help. But now that the worker is aware of the problem she is hopeful that she will be able to con-vince the older woman to apply for the available funds.

-×-

June Doyle is eighty-five and has been widowed for twenty years. Her husband was a factory worker and left her with very little money. She lives on Social Security, which is not sufficient to take care of extra expenses such as the upkeep of her home. She lives in a brick two-story corner row house. It has a living room, dining room, and kitchen on the first floor and three bedrooms and a bath upstairs.

Because she had not been able to pay for needed repairs over the past ten years the house was in a state of disrepair, both inside and outside. The local outreach worker had become aware of her situ-ation. He visited June and told her about the funding programs that were available to her. She was delighted to learn about these pro-grams since she had been very unhappy with the condition of her house but did not know what to do. The outreach worker helped her apply to the local housing agency which was a participant in the HUD small cities rehabilitation program. The agency was able to give Mrs. Doyle $8,000 worth of repairs on her house. They replaced the furnace and the front and back doors, and put in new windows on the first floor and in the basement. Inside, they replas-tered and painted some of the rooms and replaced floors that were rotten.

The HUD small cities rehabilitation program is designed to help stabilize decaying neighborhoods. Unfortunately, this excellent pro-gram is only available in certain parts of the country. For those homeowners whose income falls within specified limits, the money for repairs is given as a grant, and does not have to be repaid unless the house is sold within a specified period of time after the repairs are completed. If the applicant is over the income limit, he or she is still eligible to receive funds in the form of a low-interest loan.

Dorothy Barlow, a widow of many years, is a hale and hearty seventy-four. She was only married for a short time and was not particularly happy as a married person. She said, "I didn't care for marriage. It was too confining for me." Dorothy is a free spirit and a "no nonsense" kind of person. For over thirty years she worked as a bookkeeper and systems analyst for an engineering firm in a large city. When her job became too routine she quit and went into business for herself. For the next fifteen years she set up bookkeeping systems for small businesses. "I prefer my independence. I'm suited for freedom," she explained.

She retired from her own business twelve years ago. At that time she was living in a small apartment in the city, but she wanted to move to a rural area where she could own a house, garden, and work with a hammer and saw. She found a house that was advertised in the newspaper, looked at it, and discovered that it really met all her needs. "It was small and very cheap. It needed a lot of work, so it would give me a chance to do carpentry and other repairs. It was in the country but close to shopping and the bus so I wouldn't be isolated. And it was all on one floor. I didn't want to have to climb stairs as I got older," she explained.

The house was indeed in a very run-down condition. It had originally been used as a farmstand and was later enlarged to include a kitchen. The house has an eat-in kitchen, living room, and small bedroom and bath. Because it is so compact it is very inexpensive to heat. This is important to Dorothy because she lives on Social Security and her limited savings.

Aside from paying for a new roof and plumbing repairs in the bathroom, she did everything herself, including plastering, painting, and building cabinets in the kitchen and living room. She said that she thoroughly enjoyed this work and looked upon it as a hobby. Dorothy showed me the improvements to her house with a great deal of pride. Since her particular interest is carpentry, she has been working for the past few summers tearing down a woodshed and moving it to another location. She did this to give herself more patio space. She is still completing the new shed and seems to really need this type of physical activity.

During the cold weather in late fall, winter, and early spring, she is confined more to the inside of her home where she spends her time crocheting afghans and reading historical novels. She said, "I never have enough time to do all the reading I would like." She seems to enjoy the winters even though she cannot be outdoors. "I feel a sense of peacefulness in the winter."

Dorothy is a loner, but she is also a very intelligent and knowledgeable person and has familiarized herself with the various local and county services for the elderly. She takes advantage of the free county medical mobile unit that comes to her area twice a year and gets a medical examination that includes a blood pressure checkup. Every two months canned goods are made available free to low-income people at a food distribution center in the county and Dorothy frequetly takes advantage of this program.

She also used a homemaking service when she was housebound recovering from a broken ankle. She did not use this service for very long: being the independent person that she is, she borrowed a neighbor's chair that rolled on casters and used it to wheel herself around the house.

She uses the county transportation service for seniors at least once a week to shop for food and other items in the nearby shopping centers. She recognizes the importance of some social contact and has joined a club that meets once a week at a neighbor's home. But she adds, "I don't get too involved because I like my freedom and my privacy."

When Dorothy first moved to her new home twelve years ago she needed some extra income to help defray the cost of the initial repairs on the house. Through the Green Thumb Program she found a part-time job working twenty hours a week as the village clerk-treasurer. She claimed that she had to put in more time each week because "the records were in such a mess." She enjoyed part of her job, particularly attending the town board meetings which were held once a month. After three years she decided to leave. "I felt like I had a job again and I wanted to be retired. It took up too much time." Also, with the money she had earned, she had been able to pay for some of the work that needed to be done to fix up the house.

About six years ago, the foundation of the house began to rot. Worse, dirt and rocks from the steep incline behind her house started sliding down toward the house. Fortunately, she discovered a federal program sponsored by the United States Department of

Housing and Urban Development (HUD) that gave grants to income-eligible people for major repairs. In her area this program was administered by the Rural Ulster Preservation Company (RUPCO).

The funding agency first evaluated her income eligibility. After determining that she met their guidelines they inspected the house and decided what needed to be done. They hired the contractors and supervised the job. Dorothy's house required major changes in order to make it livable. To prevent the land on the hill in the back from sliding toward the house they built a sturdy retaining wall. Since the house was heated by inadequate and dangerous kerosene heaters, they installed electric baseboard heat. This system was the most efficient and the least expensive to maintain because natural gas was not available in her area.

Dorothy was overjoyed about the renovations to her house. She said, "I really love it and can live here quite comfortably now. I wish this program was available when I first moved in and I would not have felt that I was 'camping out.'" It is likely that Dorothy would not have been able to continue living in her house without these repairs.

In addition to the RUPCO program she also found a weatherization program administered by a county housing committee for seniors. They cut a window in the attic for ventilation, installed new windows with storms, and put insulation in the outside walls. "Now the house is real warm in the winter and cool in the summer. Without this winterization and the help from HUD I would have had to move out in the winter months. All these programs make a big difference to a low-income senior," she added.

Dorothy has also made a few changes on the inside of her house to make it a safer place to live. (See next chapter for further discussion of these safety devices.) She covered the bathroom floor with a rug, to make it safer to walk on with wet feet; she installed a grab bar on the wall next to the bathtub; and she pasted a nonslip floor in the bathtub.

She continues to enjoy her home and her life-style and likes doing service for her community. When she finishes rebuilding the shed she plans to volunteer at the local historical museum. She has served on the grand jury, and twice on the petit jury.

Dorothy enjoys cooking and says that she invites a friend for dinner once or twice a week. She also eats dinner out every Thursday and Sunday.

"My home is so important to me. I enjoy my independence. Home means happiness—to be able to have a little garden for growing some herbs and vegetables, to sit on my patio, to hammer and saw outside, and to feel free to do whatever I want. In a senior citizen residence, you are not free to do these things," she said as she summed up her feelings about staying in her own house.

There are loans and grants on a federal level to promote sound community development and safe and sanitary housing. Major funding is provided through community development block grants, which serve metropolitan cities and urban counties, and the Farmers Home Administration, which services rural areas—these areas "include open country and places with population of 10,000 or less and under certain conditions, towns and cities between 10,000 and 20,000 population."[2] These programs are usually administered through state or local agencies.

The Community Development Block Grant program allows for many kinds of community development, among which is neighborhood revitalization. Funds provided to restore blighted areas by such means as housing repairs helped June Doyle, as we saw earlier. A minimum of 60 percent of these funds must be spent on low- and moderate-income people. This money is allocated to counties and cities based on a specific formula.

The Farmers Home Administration has two major programs: section 502 and section 504. The former provides loans to low- and moderate-income people for housing construction, purchases, and repairs. The latter assists those with very low incomes to repair or improve their homes. Loans are granted at the extremely low rate of 1 percent interest; if the potential recipient is sixty-two or older and has insufficient income to pay back the loan, the loan becomes a grant.

Federal money is also available for weatherization assistance. Funds are distributed by the federal Energy and Health and Human Services departments to the states. In New Jersey the Weatherization Assistance Program uses federal funds to assist low- to moderate-income people in making their homes more energy-efficient. Heating system improvement and insulation services such as caulking, weather stripping, window and door repair or replacement are provided free of charge.

The weatherization program that helped Dorothy Barlow received some of its funds from federal sources. Called the Shandaken

Revitalization Plan (SHARP), it provides all the services described above at no charge. The program is available to all income-eligible people, and is open to renters as well as homeowners. With SHARP's help, elderly homeowners increase the warmth of their homes while reducing heating costs. Weatherization repairs often have the added benefit of making the older person feel safer and more secure.[3]

The Home Energy Assistance Program (HEAP) is a fourth federal housing program designed to help low-income persons meet home heating costs. This program provides money for heating bills. Senior citizens sixty years of age or older may apply for benefits by mail; all other people must apply in person. Payments vary depending on the size of the household, the amount of income, and the type of heating system. HEAP is usually administered by state departments of energy.

Many different housing programs are offered throughout the country by state and local governments. New York State, for example, offers the Residential Emergency Service to Offer Repairs for the Elderly (RESTORE). This program makes grants through municipal action groups to homeowners who are sixty years of age or older and who fall within specified income limits. Each eligible homeowner can receive up to $5,000 for repairs.

New Jersey's Lifeline Credit Program offers utility assistance to persons sixty-five years or older. The program is restricted to persons of low income. The recipients receive a yearly grant of $225 for their gas and/or electric bills.

The Area on Aging Agency in Jasper, Texas, offers a one-time grant for the elderly for critical repairs. The agency uses volunteer labor and can't afford to make expensive repairs, but with its limited resources it has been able to help more than 130 homeowners by repairing floors, stairs, roofs, and plumbing.[4]

In addition to assistance for major repairs and renovations that may be necessary to enable older people to remain in their own homes, it is important for them to have help with minor repairs and chore services. These services are usually sponsored locally. Many use volunteers, including the elderly themselves, many of whom used to make their livings as plumbers, etc. These repair services have names like Chore Service, Mr. Fixit, and Mr. Handyman.

A county handyman service in the northeast uses volunteers from industry, retiree organizations, and churches. In addition to making minor repairs, this handyman service also offers help with yard-work. The workers range in age from their early twenties to their late seventies. "It is so hard to find someone to fix a small thing like a kitchen faucet or a lamp. I'm so grateful to the handyman service for their help," says one elderly widow. The volunteers also reap rewards from being a part of this program. One young man said, "I get to know many older people and it makes me feel like I have lots of grandparents."

A Mr. Fixit service in the Midwest was housed in a senior center so the news of its existence traveled quickly in the community. Greta, a seventy-eight-year-old divorcee, lived in a one-bedroom apartment. She was a proud and independent person and had no family except for a few nieces and nephews who lived in Canada. She had been a participant at the senior center for eleven years. She is extremely arthritic and has had two knee replacements. She is able to walk but needs the aid of a three-pronged cane.

Through a federal employment program (see chapter 6) she obtained a clerical position at the borough hall where she works twenty hours a week in the tax office. This job was very important to her because she needed the extra income. She worked for five years but had to give it up when her physical condition worsened.

Greta said, "'Mr. Fixit' has been a life-saver for me. I don't know how I would manage my home and my life without all the things he did for me. And it was all free. I didn't have to pay for anything except a few pieces of wood." The program provided many services for her, such as repairing her appliances and some of the old furniture. In addition, the volunteer adjusted her toilet seat, and made an intermediate step to the porch stairs so that she could get up and down more easily. "But the most wonderful thing he did for me was to make me a very light high stool with a short back. He chained it to my outside railing. Now I can sit while I wait for the bus. You see, I can't stand for very long, so this little stool was a godsend!" she said joyfully.

Laura, another divorcee in her early seventies, owned a dilapidated house. Although she was extremely frail, she was determined not to move. She learned of the Mr. Fixit program through a neighbor who attended the senior center.

She could not open and close her windows; the volunteer repairman replaced the sash cords, and her windows worked again. He repaired her air conditioning unit and placed it in the window. He shortened her cane, which had been too tall for her to use properly. He put grab bars in the bathroom and repaired the steps to the basement. He provided weather stripping and caulking on the doors and windows. His visits didn't end after he made the most critical repairs. Whenever she needed light bulbs replaced, he was there to do the job. "And now I have someone to put in my screens in the spring and my storm windows in the fall. He also hangs my draperies in the winter and takes them down in the summer. My house looks so much nicer now and it's so much more comfortable," Laura said. Without this kind of assistance it is difficult to imagine that Laura could have continued to live in her own home.

A more extensive volunteer program exists in Tacoma, Washington. It is sponsored by Catholic Community Services and is called the Volunteer Chore Program. In addition to helping with yardwork and minor repairs, this group provides assistance with housework, cooking, laundry, personal care, errands or shopping, and limited companionship. It is staffed by volunteers. There is no charge for the service but clients can make donations. As one client commented, "I don't know what I would do without my chore help. I sure couldn't do it myself." But clients are not the only beneficiaries of the program.

"I am 68 and I have been by myself for two years after my wife died. . . . I would like to be doing something for someone else. Besides, without love, what is there left?" said one of the volunteers.[5]

Throughout the United States there are programs and services to assist older people with repairs, renovations, and chore services in order to help them remain in their own homes. Many of these programs are designed specifically to aid low- and moderate-income elderly. Some provide outright grants while others issue low interest loans. And even for those seniors who are outside the income guidelines, there is help with hiring competent and reliable contractors.

In addition to the above services, there are some adjustments which can be made to the home to make it more comfortable and less accident-prone. I will be exploring this topic in the next chapter.

A Stitch in Time

How to Make the Home More Secure and Safer

Although repairs and renovations are necessary for the homes of some of the elderly, modifications to accommodate the aging process are needed in the homes of many more aging people. These modifications can greatly increase the safety and security of the home.

Increasing Home Security

A relatively new state program in New Jersey is concerned with making the home more secure. Called the Senior Citizens Security Housing and Transportation Program, it is available free to any person who is sixty years old or older. Although this type of service may not be available in every state right now, federal legislation has just been introduced that, if passed, will create a similar national program.

The New Jersey program does not have any income restrictions, but does give priority to low-income and minority groups residing in high-crime areas. Its purpose is to provide increased security to homeowners and renters. Administered by the area agency on aging, and usually implemented through the local police department's crime prevention unit, the program offers intercom systems, replacement of doors, door and window locks and frames, door glazing, peep holes, better security for mailboxes, improved external lighting, and automatic timers for outside lights.[1] In addition to responding to requests for safety devices, the police also conduct housing security surveys to identify measures that would make residences more secure.

In one county in New Jersey during one year the crime prevention unit helped over 900 elderly people. These people lived in one of eight towns that had been identified as high-crime areas. The program allows $200 as a maximum cost for materials per home; since the police purchase needed materials in bulk they are able to install all the safety devices for this amount or less. This police unit also gives free lectures on crime prevention. They instruct older people about how to cut down hedges so that burglars cannot easily hide behind them; how to identify suspicious people; how to recognize potential "scams"; and how to keep pocketbooks and wallets well hidden in the house.

A seventy-two-year-old widow was involved in a scam. A woman with a young child knocked on her door and asked if they could come in because the child was not feeling well and needed a glass of water. The widow went into the kitchen and got a glass of water for the youngster. After the woman and child left, the widow discovered that her handbag, containing all her money and the only set of house keys she had, was missing. She called a locksmith, who told her that it would cost $60 each to replace the front and back door locks. Unable to pay for new locks, she was so frightened at the thought that this woman would return and rob her when she was away that she never left her house and did not sleep at night, but dozed sitting up in a chair during the day. Since she was not friendly with any of her neighbors she did not know where to turn for help. This went on for six days, and she gradually used up all the food she had in the house.

Fortunately, she heard a public service announcement on the radio about a new senior citizen safety program. She immediately called the police department which responded quickly and serviced her on an emergency basis. The police quickly ascertained her needs and installed two dead-bolt safety locks, placed security pins in the first-floor windows, replaced the front outside light with a new high-pressure sodium light, and put reflective house numbers on the front door. They also advised her to keep her pocketbook out of sight and cautioned her about allowing strangers into her house.

-※-

Another widow who was eighty years of age and lived in a two-story row house encountered a different type of problem which thoroughly frightened her. While she was out shopping, a young fellow on a bicycle grabbed her handbag, knocked her down, and sped away on his bike. She was able to walk home since luckily she was not hurt. However, besides losing her money, she had lost both sets of house keys when her bag was stolen. In order to get into her house she broke a back window. She telephoned the police and reported the mugging. Like the other widow, she was too fearful to leave the house. This state of affairs continued for almost five days, since she could not afford to put in new locks or repair the broken window. Fortunately, the police needed more information and sent a special crime unit to visit the widow. They told the elderly woman about the housing security program. She readily agreed to participate and said, "What a wonderful blessing! You must have been sent from heaven." The police replaced the broken pane of glass in the back window, put new locks on the front and back doors, put security pins in the first-floor windows, and gave her a new sensor front light.

⁕

A third widow, seventy-nine years of age, had lived for a long time in her present house. While she aged in place, her neighborhood deteriorated. According to the police, it was one of the worst areas in the city. It had heavy drug traffic. Parts of her house were in very bad shape but she could not afford the cost of needed repairs. She did not know where to turn for help. Fortunately, she learned about the housing security program from a neighbor.

When the police responded to her call they were amazed at the condition of her house. The doors were so rotted that they would not support any locks. They referred her to the county housing office which had funds for repairs. They replaced both the front and back doors with new doors that had peepholes and replaced all the windows that were rotted. When this work was completed, the police were able to give her new locks on the doors, security pins in the windows, and a reflective address plate on the front door. In addition, they installed a light in the back of the house which was on an alley way that had public access.

In this New Jersey county, the police are now routinely supplying each elderly household they service with a "stress" outside front light. The "stress" light works like an ordinary light when it is switched on in a regular manner. However, if the occupant is in trouble, the switch can be flicked twice which makes the light pulse on and off. This alerts patroling police to enter the house and investigate the trouble. Neighbors are informed about the special light and are told to call the police if they see it flashing.

This program has been very successful throughout New Jersey and has received a great deal of publicity. For relatively little money it has produced a safer and more secure environment for the elderly, particularly those living on small, fixed incomes. Some counties have imposed income limits on eligibility for free service, but no one is charged more than a small fee. One county uses a special team of retired police officers to conduct this safety program.

One elderly gentleman works as a part-time janitor at a local school. He had a very simple request. He needed a more secure lock and a peephole on his front door, and an outside light. When these were installed, he breathed a sigh of relief and said, "Now I feel much safer at night and when someone knocks on my door, I can see who it is. Before I had the peephole I was afraid to answer the door because I didn't know who it was."

A number of older people who had been burglarized several times could not afford to secure their homes. Through this new program they have had outside lights installed to ward off intruders, as well as double-bolt locks on their doors and safety bars on downstairs windows. Because so many of the elderly live in older homes, which often have deteriorated doors and flimsy locks, they suffer a disproportionate number of break-ins. At relatively small cost, a safe housing program can easily correct many of the safety deficiencies that make the elderly easy prey to burglars.

Increasing Home Safety

Now we need to take a look at the entire house and its furnishings to see what kind of modifications should be considered in order to make the home more livable.

We know that the fifth or sixth leading cause of death for the elderly is accidents—and 80 percent of these accidents occur in the home. Even when an accident does not result in death, it often results in permanent injury and disability. Therefore, it is important to minimize accident risk in the home. Houses are designed for couples and growing families and do not usually include the safety features that can reduce accident risk for older homeowners. As persons age they experience loss of vision, hearing, smell, and touch.

In addition, they become less stable in their gait, lose muscle strength and coordination, and experience other declines in their functional mobility. These changes are usually so gradual that they may not become noticeable to the elderly person until advanced old age.

It is important for older people to check their homes to see what kind of changes might be made to improve the quality and safety of their lives. Look around each room with an analytic eye. Even small changes can make a big difference in comfort and safety. Perhaps furniture needs to be rearranged to eliminate obstacles. Scatter rugs should be removed and replaced with skid-free floor covering. In the bathroom, consider installing a grab bar, handrails, a seat in the tub or shower, and lever handles in place of doorknobs (easier on arthritic fingers) for faucets. In the bedroom, a lamp and a telephone should be close to the bed. In the kitchen, staples and essential utensils should be stowed in low drawers and cupboards. A whistling teakettle could be useful here, too—the whistle reminds the older person to turn off the stove. Do not forget a large, well-marked calendar, a clearly printed list of important numbers posted near the telephone, a compartmentalized pill container, and any other simple memory-joggers that can help sustain a sense of self-confidence.[2]

I found that most of the people I interviewed had not thought about making any changes to their homes to accommodate their aging. A few had had studs placed in the wall next to the bathtub and installed handrails, to make getting in and out of the tub easier and safer. An older woman who had always lived alone had done this in her bathroom. She did feel that since she wanted to remain living in her own house for as long as possible, that, "I am so lucky that my house is all on one floor and I won't have to climb stairs when I am very old." (She is now seventy-four years old). She also remarked that her house was very close to shopping and transportation and this would become more important when she was no longer able to drive a car. The only other accommodation she has made to her age is to have an automatic garage opener installed since the door was becoming increasingly more difficult to manually push up and pull down. Also she felt it was safer not to have to get out of her car and walk to the garage to open it, particularly at night.

At a senior center, about a dozen older women joined in a discussion about safety in the home. A few had replaced regular shower heads with European hand-held showers. They found these much easier to use, especially for washing their hair. Another woman mentioned installing a plastic chair that sits on the broad side of the tub; this chair enables her to get into the bathtub from a sitting position. One woman had handrails installed on her basement stairs, another had put railings on her deck, a third had placed handgrips on the outside stair railing so that she could grab these when the steps were slippery. It was apparent that they had given this subject some thought but had made relatively minor adjustments in their homes.

Mr. and Mrs. Rich have been married for forty years. He is eighty-eight and she is eighty-two. They have no living family members. They live in a ranch house that has a living room, dining room, kitchen, two bedrooms, and a bath. They both are quite frail, but Mrs. Rich is in better physical condition than her husband. He is much weaker, is unstable on his feet, and uses a walker. Since the husband was having difficulty navigating the four front steps, three years ago they had a ramp installed at the entrance to the house. They changed the furniture arrangement in the living room to make a clearer path to the rest of the house. The scatter rugs in the bedroom became a hazard for Mr. Rich so these were removed and wall-to-wall carpeting was installed in their place. These were relatively simple changes but they enabled the elderly couple to move around their house with greater safety.

Their lives are also enriched by their attendance at special programs and parties at the local senior center. They receive homemaking services three days a week for two hours each day from church volunteers. A student chore service rakes the leaves, shovels the snow, and takes the air conditioners in and out of the windows according to the season. Since this couple have no family to help them, they could not continue to remain in their own home without the community support services and the changes that they made in the house.

Jerry and Peg Marsh, a couple in their eighties, live in a two-story house on an acre of land in a semirural area in the Northeast. They are both attractive, intelligent, and articulate people who had held professional jobs. Jerry had been an editor for a large publishing company and Peg had been a research librarian. Their professional interests were very much in evidence in the home since most of the rooms contained many shelves of books.

They have two daughters: one is single and lives in a city about a hundred miles away; the other is divorced and lives about three hundred miles away. They are a close family and the daughters visit as frequently as possible but obviously are not available on a day-to-day basis.

When they were working they lived in a large apartment in a big city and enjoyed all the cultural activities that were available. They began to think of their retirement and decided that they would like to live in a more rural area and have a house large enough to accommodate their mutual interests and extensive book collection. Twenty-two years ago they found a small vacation home that had the potential for expansion since it was on a large piece of land.

While they were employed they used the house for vacations and occasional weekends. After retirement they gave up their city apartment and moved to their rural home. At the time, only the first floor of the house was finished; the second floor was an unfinished attic. The first floor had a kitchen, a small dining-living room, a study, and a small bedroom and bath. While this space had been adequate as a vacation home, it was too small to satisfy their needs as a permanent place to live.

They decided to finish the attic and convert it into a master bedroom and bath. There was enough space to make it into a very large room with two walls of bookshelves and two walk-in closets. Since they needed a fire exit they added an outside staircase. Since at that time Jerry and Peg were already well into their 70s and both came from long-lived families, they began to think of their old age. "Peg is the planner in our family," Jerry said. "I just go along from day to day and don't really think about the future." Peg added, "I think that men have more denial and that women tend to be more realistic."

Although they are both in relatively good health, Jerry did have a coronary by-pass operation five years ago, and Peg has diabetes, slightly elevated cholesterol, and high blood pressure. They remain very active, however, and continue to drive and to take long walks for exercise. Peg had decided to study the violin and began to take lessons six years ago. She enjoys this very much and meets with two other amateur musicians regularly to play chamber trios.

They spend their time reading, listening to music, watching TV, and writing. They entertain frequently and have many overnight guests. As Peg puts it, "We have a steady stream of visitors in the summer and we love it."

Although Jerry is retired he still attends national publishing conferences, and has recently returned from attending a convention on the West coast. He also still serves on the board of a professional magazine and writes occasional articles for it. Since he lives in an "arty" community, he has been asked to lead a book discussion group. He was delighted to take up this new challenge and has been actively involved with several different groups over the past few years.

Peg had begun to think about the suitability of their present housing in light of their recent health problems. Without discussing this concern with her husband she started to explore other living arrangements for the elderly. When she found an attractive life-care community (see chapter 10) she told Jerry about it and he agreed to take a look at it. Neither of them thought it made any sense for them at this stage of their life. "The apartments were so small," Jerry said. "And where would we keep all our books? We would be cut off from family and friends since we would no longer have the room to have them stay overnight." Peg added, "I don't know how I'd like living with only old people. They looked so frail. Now we have many friends who are younger and very vital and this helps keep us stimulated and active."

Since their preference was to remain in their own home for as long as possible, they decided to reassess the house and see if they could make any changes that would ensure their continued occupancy. Peg assigned herself this task. With her library background she knew that catalogues must exist on special devices for the elderly. She began reading these catalogues and discovered some simple changes that could be made in the kitchen and bathroom. She replaced the shower head with a hand-held shower, had two grab bars installed on the bathtub walls, and added another grab bar next to the toilet. In the kitchen, she had a carpenter build shelves under the cabinets so that she could reach the everyday dishes and utensils without having to stand on a ladder.

Peg and Jerry began to think about some longer range needs when they could no longer drive or do their own cooking, shopping, or housework. They felt that the upstairs bedroom and bath were large enough to be converted into a studio apartment at some future date, at which time they would move downstairs. In the meantime, they felt they could use an addition to the house since they had outgrown their tiny living room and wanted a larger space for entertaining and for Jerry's discussion groups.

Jerry and Peg both had Social Security and good pensions so that they could afford to make an addition to their house. They hired an architect and had a glass-enclosed room and a small bath added at the back of the house. This addition overlooks the garden and they spend many pleasant hours there. It has also provided more wall space for their growing book collection.

Peg, the family planner, commented, "When we reach that time in life that we need extra help in the house, we won't have to consider moving in with children or leaving our lovely home. We will be able to hire a couple and let them live rent-free in the upstairs unit, while we can move downstairs and use our new addition as a master bedroom. It should work out well since then we will not have to climb any stairs. The couple can drive us to visit friends and attend concerts and theater so that we won't be socially isolated in our old age. We think that this would be better than a move to a special residence for the elderly."

However, they both agreed that their present living arrangement would have to be revaluated if one of them dies (see chapter 10).

Martha Haines, an eighty-nine-year-old widow, lives in a ranch house. Her husband had owned his own heating fuel business and she had been an elementary schoolteacher. Her husband died twenty-five years ago. She has two sons, both of whom are married. One lives on the West coast, and the other lives next door to her. This son's wife works and unfortunately there is not a good relationship between Martha and her daughter-in-law.

Martha is an intelligent woman and until her recent bout with crippling arthritis led a very active and independent life. Clothes are very important to her and she is always meticulously dressed. Her home is spotless and she obviously takes great pride in how both she and her house look.

She enjoys reading but her eyesight has deteriorated so that she can only read the large-print daily newspaper. She uses talking books and listens to the radio. In addition to arthritis she suffers from diabetes. She is able to give herself the necessary injections. Her mobility has become limited so that she requires the use of a walker.

Martha was determined to stay in her house because it gave her so much pleasure. She particularly enjoyed sitting in her sunporch in the morning sun and looking out at the garden. But this was becoming increasingly difficult for her because she had to navigate one step to enter the porch. She realized that she had other problems in getting around her house and asked her son to help her solve them.

Together, mother and son looked at the problem areas in the house and decided to hire a carpenter who could design appropriate solutions that would not be too costly. Luckily they found a recently retired workman who was willing to do the job for a little more than the cost of the materials. The first change he made was to build a small ramp from the kitchen to the sunporch so that Martha could use her walker between the two rooms. The carpenter also widened the door to the bathroom to accommodate the walker. He put grab bars on either side of the toilet to aid Martha in getting on and off; he replaced the bathtub with a wide stall shower that had a plastic seat and also installed a grab bar in the shower. He added a railing in the hallway to give Martha extra support in walking between the rooms. The carpenter built a high counter in the kitchen and a bar stool with a back so that she could eat all her meals there.

Martha was very pleased with the modifications to her house and showed them off with real pride to everyone who visited. "Look how beautiful the work is and how nicely it all fits in," she said. "And it looks like it's always been here. Now I can live in my house forever and never have to leave!"

-✳-

Ruby, a sixty-seven-year-old widow, broke both her legs when she fell while stepping off a curb. Hospitalized, she required three operations. She spent the next three months in a nursing home while she was recuperating and receiving physical therapy. She was eager to return home but she could not manage the return without extensive home-care services. In addition, she would have been confined to her room. Since she was a very independent person, she did not like this arrangement or the other alternative of remaining at the nursing home for an indefinite period.

She conferred with her son and daughter-in-law who were very sympathetic and wanted their mother to be able to return home. They asked the hospital social worker to help them figure out what needed to be done in their mother's house to enable her to live safely by herself.

Ruby's son and his wife made the necessary changes in the house while she was still at the nursing home. They placed railings on either side of the entrance stairs (there were three steps to climb to enter), and rounded off the one step and added a short handrail at the back door. Inside the house, they rearranged the furniture to allow for a safe and easy path through the rooms with a walker and replaced the scatter rugs with wall-to-wall carpeting. The kitchen required nothing more complicated than a rearrangement of the items in the cupboards so that the dishes and food that were used most often were readily accessible. The bathroom needed the most extensive alterations. Here they had to install handrails around the tub and on either side of the toilet, buy a plastic seat for the bathtub, put in a hand-held shower head, and buy a raised seat for the toilet.

Not only did these simple changes allow Ruby to return home for her long recuperation but the doctor felt that her house was now much safer and would greatly reduce the chance of accidents.

-×-

Marion, a married woman of sixty-five, had a near-fatal automobile accident several years ago. The van she was driving was hit by a tractor-trailer truck that was traveling at a very high speed. Her van careened off the road and crashed into a house. Practically all the bones in the lower part of her body were broken and she also suffered some internal injuries.

These physical injuries were only part of the problem. She had always been a very independent person who was able to cope very well with adversity. But the trauma of this accident pushed her into anger and depression. Her daughter, who is a social worker, realized that this negative emotional state was not only bad for her but would also interfere with her physical recovery.

Marion had been widowed at an early age and had to bring up

her three children by herself. She became a schoolteacher and ended up as chairman of a high school science department before she retired five years ago. Seven years before her retirement she married again. Her second husband is a retired marine engineer and is well fixed financially. They have been able to lead a very full life. They attend the theater, visit museums, and travel extensively throughout the United States and Europe. They are both avid readers and bridge players.

Since both her brother and her older sister lived far away Sue had to assume sole responsibility for her mother. Marion's husband was seventy-two-years-old and was unable to handle his wife's depression. However, since he had sufficient funds to pay for any major modifications in the house, he was more than willing to undertake any alterations that would enable his wife to function at home. He was only too happy to have Sue take charge of this task.

Sue began by having several conferences with the rehabilitation worker at the center where her mother was receiving physical therapy. They discussed Marion's serious mobility problems and what kind of alterations to her home would be necessary to accommodate her condition. Sue learned that her mother's healing process could take a year or more and she tried to mentally prepare her mother for this long recovery period.

Sue began contacting carpenters and finally found one who understood the situation and seemed up to the task. The bathroom needed changes such as a shower stall with a seat and grab bars, grab bars on each side of the toilet, and a raised seat on the toilet. The kitchen needed to be completely redesigned. All the counters were raised so that Marion could work in a standing position. The cabinets were lowered so that she could reach the first and second shelves easily. The microwave oven was also lowered, and the kitchen floor was recovered with an industrial-type carpet so she would not slip.

All the outlets in the house were raised so that they could be reached without bending. Ramps with railings were installed at the front and back entrances. Furniture was rearranged to create a better circulation pattern throughout the house. Finally, the downstairs den was converted into a bedroom so that she would not be a prisoner on the second floor.

In addition to changes that had to be made in the house, Marion required home health aides around the clock. Her husband was very supportive and he assisted with the nursing care in any way he could. Her friends rallied around her and she had company and phone calls on a regular basis. It took her a long time to recover emotionally from the trauma, but after almost a year she was able to manage her own life again.

Ruby and Marion suffered serious injuries that necessitated major changes in their home environments. But many of the changes that enabled Ruby and Marion to make successful returns to their homes would also be useful for other elderly persons with less severe physical problems. Unfortunately, few, if any, programs exist to provide funds for these kinds of modifications. A reverse mortgage line-of-credit, however, could be used to finance any safety renovations.

A program sponsored by the area agency on aging in Charlottesville, Virginia, is specifically designed to assist people over the age of sixty in assessing the changes needed in their homes in order to improve their functioning. It targets those elderly with cognitive deficits and sensory impairments. An occupational therapist visits the home and makes an assessment of what kind of difficulties the older person is experiencing and what can be done to correct these difficulties. Volunteers make the required changes and supply appropriate safety equipment on a long-term loan basis. The area agency has also produced a video tape and a manual on how homes can be changed to meet specific functional needs of older people.[3]

For improved safety in the home, I suggest you check the following excellent references: (1) *Safety for Older Consumers: Home Safety Checklist*, and (2) *The Do.Able Renewable Home* (see footnotes for resources). I have adapted some of their suggestions to create the following check-lists.

Housewide

Electrical

1. Check all wiring and plugs for fraying and other damage
2. Keep wires out of traffic flow to prevent tripping

3. Try not to use extension cords
4. Do not place furniture or rugs over wiring
5. Raise electrical outlets 18 to 24 inches off the floor
6. Make sure all areas are well lit

Floors

1. Make sure all rugs and carpets are slip resistant
2. Check for surface irregularities—broken tiles, loose boards, etc.—and eliminate them
3. Remove raised doorway sills wherever possible
4. Avoid coating floors with slippery substances

Security

1. Locate and test smoke detectors
2. Review fire exit procedures
3. Check doors and windows for ease of opening and closing
4. Install locks where needed

In the Kitchen

1. Be sure stove and ventilation system are in good order
2. Keep paper and cloth, including loose-fitting clothing, away from the hot stove
3. Have sufficient light over work areas
4. Use lower shelves to store everyday dishes and utensils
5. Use a step stool, preferably with a handrail, to reach higher shelves

In the Bedroom

1. Keep a nightlight on in the room or in an adjacent hallway
2. Have a lamp or wall switch within reach of the bed
3. Install an extension phone next to the bed
4. Keep a flashlight handy in case of power outages; check batteries periodically
5. Keep any potential fire hazards (ashtrays, hot plates, heaters) far away from bedding—burns and mattress-related fires are leading causes of accidental death among older people

In the Bathroom

1. Provide nonskid floors in tub or shower
2. Attach securely at least one grab bar (two, if possible) to the wall of the tub, or use specially designed bars that grip the edge of the tub
3. Place a small plastic seat with a nonslip bottom in the tub or shower. (A convenient device when taking sitdown showers is a European-type shower head that can be clamped to the wall or held in the hand)
4. Remember: shower stalls are safer than tubs because of the potential for a fall when stepping over the rim of the tub—even with grab bars
5. Attach grab bars to the wall or walls alongside the toilet commode, or use a free-standing set of grab bars that fit around the commode

Halls and Stairs

1. Be sure these areas are well lit with light bulbs of sufficient wattage. (Frosted bulbs reduce glare)
2. Install light switches at the top and bottom of the stairwell
3. Guild sturdy handrails on both sides of the staircase
4. Check stair carpeting for tight fit and for rips or tears[4]

Although a variety of modifications can be introduced in older people's homes, the most useful are relatively simple and inexpensive to install. Extra handrails on staircases, grab bars alongside the toilet and bathtub, and a hand-held shower are not very costly, but contribute significantly to reducing accidents. In addition to changes in the home, many tools and devices can make life much easier for an older person. Some appliance manufacturers have developed braille overlays for control panels on their stoves and ovens; special knob covers and knob turners for stove controls for persons with arthritis; special kitchen shelf organizers; clips for easier opening of refrigerator and freezer doors; kitchen equipment designed for one-hand operations; plastic labels to mark appliance controls (see references and chapter 11).

At the beginning of this chapter I mentioned the flashing front lights that can alert neighbors or police to problems inside an elderly person's home. Before we leave the topic of safety and security I would like to familiarize my readers with some other alert systems.

For the elderly person living alone, particularly one at-risk medically, a security alarm system can be a great comfort. These systems enable a person at home to summon help in an emergency. One such system, the Life Safety System, works at the press of an emergency button, which sounds an alarm at the local fire department. Other medical-alert devices are operated through local hospitals. A home transmitter signals the hospital operator when a button on the wristband or pendant is pressed. These devices have recently been improved to allow voice communication with the operator as long as the person who needs help is within fifty feet of the telephone.

A carrier-alert program sponsored by the U.S. Postal Service monitors individuals who sign up for the service; the mail carrier checks each day to see if the previous day's mail has been removed from the box. In addition, volunteer organizations in many communities maintain telephone reassurance services for elderly people registered with them (see chapter 6).[5]

Enhancing Independence

*Available Community Services and Programs
to Maintain the Elderly in Their Own Homes*

In addition to being able to manage one's own home financially
and physically it is important to know what services and programs
exist in the community to enable one to cope with the aging process
while remaining independent. These programs range over many
areas: telephone reassurance, friendly visiting, Outreach, legal services, Meals-on-Wheels, home health aides, transportation and es-
cort services, senior centers, adult day care, educational and volunteer opportunities, employment, and recreation.

Many surveys have been made to determine the use of community services. Unfortunately, these surveys indicate that a significant
number of older people and their families are either unaware of
services available to them or wait until a crisis develops before at-
tempting to find out what does exist. It makes much more sense to
look ahead and become familiar with the community programs that
could serve your needs now or in the future, so that you do not
have to start locating the proper help when you're already in a
stressful situation. In addition, these community resources could
make a big difference in your day-to-day life by enabling you to
continue to follow your own life-style and improve the quality of
your life.

Companionship and Support Services

A number of different programs offer companionship and support
services. One of the best known is Friendly Visiting. A good ex-

ample of this kind of program is called Home Friends. It has been in existence for over two years and uses 60 volunteers. These helpers range from young mothers with children who visit in the daytime to working people who visit in the evenings or on weekends, to retirees.

Madge Green, a widow, is 80 years old. She had to leave school at age eleven because her mother became very ill and Madge was needed to run the household. Madge married young and never worked outside the home. Her husband had a blue-collar job. She has lived in her present house all her married life. It has two stories and looks like a doll's house. There are three small rooms on the first floor and two bedrooms and a bath upstairs. The side yard has a white marble birdbath, a fountain, and a beautiful garden. Gardening is her main interest; she obviously takes great pride in her flowers and plants.

Madge has been widowed a long time and finds living alone very lonely. She has always been a very passive person socially. Her brothers and sisters are dead but her two sons are very caring; one lives far away but the other one lives in the next town.

Madge is a diabetic and takes insulin. More recently she has developed arthritis. She is an avid walker and also enjoys handwork. Her only other activity is attending church, which she does almost daily. She has very few friends, is not a joiner, and refuses to attend a nearby senior center. She also will not consider sharing her house with a stranger. Madge needs on-going emotional support that her sons cannot supply.

Her younger son learned of the Home Friends program and told his mother about it. She agreed to contact them and ask for a friendly visitor. Fortunately, the agency was able to find Irene, a fifty-year-old married woman from the same ethnic background as Madge. Irene and Madge hit it off very well and Irene has been seeing Madge for the past year and a half. Irene visits Madge at least once a week and spends a few hours with her each time. Most of the time Irene takes her out. They have lunch together at a restaurant, or attend flower shows. Madge looks forward to these outings and seems to be less depressed or lonely.

A Chore and Companionship Program run by a public high school in a large suburb in the Northeast offers a variation of friendly visiting. Part of an intergenerational program that provides services to the elderly and brings young people and seniors together, Chore and Companionship was an outgrowth of a youth employment service that has been in existence for more than twenty-five years.

The Chore and Companionship program was started seven years ago and has been very successful. It was originally funded by a private foundation and run by volunteers. It now has a paid director, one of whose responsibilities is to organize an annual fund-raising drive. She hopes that the town will help with financing since the program operates on a relatively small budget.

Students are hired at $3.50 to $4.00 an hour, and usually work two hours a week. The older recipients are expected to pay the students' wages, but if they cannot afford the regular rate they pay only $1.00 an hour and the program pays the rest. The student and the older person make their own arrangements about how many hours the student will work. The students assist the elderly with household chores but usually become companions in the process. The goal of the program is not to supply inexpensive maid-service, but rather to maintain frail elderly people in their homes and to provide the opportunity for young and old to develop meaningful relationships.

The students are carefully screened for this program and need a recommendation from a teacher or a counselor. Thirty students are currently working; each is trained and monitored by the director. The students have the choice of participating and earning money for their work or receiving five credits a year from their school for community service. If they choose the latter option, they must meet with the director once a week, keep a journal, and write a final report on their experience.

Most of the students do light housework, laundry, yardwork, and run errands. The students read to the visually impaired and do any writing that is required. They also may balance checkbooks. Another hundred volunteers—mostly high school and college students—shovel snow and rake leaves for those elderly unable to perform these tasks. The program is a splendid success at doing what it was designed to do: the elderly receive needed services for little cost, the students earn money or school credit, and both groups benefit from their interaction.

Sylvia Reed, an eighty-year-old widow, lived in a one-bedroom apartment. She had several medical conditions, including diabetes and circulatory problems. She had difficulty standing and needed help with her household chores. Her two children, a daughter who lived far away and a son who lived nearby, were obviously unable to help her during the day. Her son did do the weekly food shopping with her.

She learned about the Chore and Companionship program and applied for a student helper. Carey, a seventeen-year-old senior at the high school, worked for Sylvia until she graduated. Carey did the housework and took the laundry to the basement laundry room. She also did some food shopping for Sylvia. Sylvia taught Carey how to knit and they spent many pleasant hours together talking and visiting.

Sylvia was partially homebound but did manage to get to the senior center on occasion. Outside of family, Carey was Sylvia's main visitor. They formed a very close relationship. After Carey left for college, she continued to write, telephone, and visit Sylvia. "Without my little friend, I could not continue to live in my apartment. I don't know how I would have managed without her," she said.

The problems of a couple in their mid-80s demonstrate the value of programs such as Chore and Companionship. The husband was extremely ill, but he did not need hospital care. He did need to be assisted in getting in and out of bed. His wife was unable to help him, so he would sleep sitting up in his chair. After a student was assigned to this couple, he came five days a week and would help the elderly man transfer from the bed to the chair each morning and back from the chair to the bed at night (on weekends, a daughter was able to perform this task for her father). This small service allowed the man, sick as he was, to continue living with his wife and to die in his own bed. The program records many such success stories. Another example: a widow in her nineties was able to forestall entering a nursing home for a year because of the help she received from a high school student.

Once a student enrolls in the program he or she tends to remain for the duration of the high school years. The students learn about the aging process, its myths and realities, and older people's strengths and weaknesses. The program not only introduces the students to the field of gerontology but also gives them the feeling of satisfaction that comes with public service. Real friendships develop between the young and the old, much like loving grandparents and grandchildren. When a student left the program because of college or work, there was a real sense of loss for both the student and the person(s) he or she helped.

Outreach Services

One of the less-known services available in most areas is called Outreach. Instead of the elderly person seeking help by contacting an agency, the Outreach service contacts the senior and offers assistance—either over the telephone or more often by visiting the person in the home. Outreach workers tend to be older people themselves who are trained and supervised by social workers or other community agency staff. They receive minimum wage and work twenty hours a week.

Betty and John, a very elderly couple, have lived in a one-bedroom apartment for thirty years. They have two very devoted children, a son and a daughter, who live in the area. However, these children both have full-time jobs and large families and can offer only limited help to their parents. The hospital social worker contacted the local Outreach service and requested an aide visit and help for the elderly couple.

The Outreach aide spent a long time with Betty and John on her first visit. She found that they both had serious medical problems and functional disabilities. Five years ago John had a stroke and now walks with a cane, is somewhat disoriented, and is quite demanding. His wife was in fairly good shape until he became ill, but she then developed Piaget's disease which caused mobility problems and made her very depressed. She uses a walker. Both people are essentially homebound. Betty's illness caused a role reversal with her husband since he became the caretaker for his wife and took responsibility for most household tasks.

It was obvious that this elderly couple could not continue to remain in their own apartment without a great deal of outside help. The aide connected them with a community senior volunteer service, which provides food shopping once a week. A homemaker was hired to do the household cleaning and to assist the couple with personal care, such as getting in and out of the bathtub. A Mr. Fixit volunteer (see chapter 4) came to the house and installed grab bars around the tub, loosened windows that were stuck or difficult to open and shut, and changed light bulbs whenever it was necessary. There were no fees for any of these services. In addition to providing the couple with all this assistance, the Outreach aide visited them on a regular basis two or three times a week. She felt that many visits were necessary in view of their emotional problems. Betty and John were able to remain living in their own home, despite the severity of their handicaps, because of the community services they received and the friendly visiting and socialization provided by the Outreach service.

Outreach aides have helped many older people find the help that they need. A widow in her mid-eighties had lived in a house for a long period of time. She had become somewhat confused, disoriented, and frail. Her only son lived thirty miles away. She needed companionship and help with housework and cooking.

A homemaker who did the cooking, shopping, and housework and also provided companionship was hired. The son paid for this service. One homemaker worked five days a week from 10 A.M. to noon and another from 7 to 11 P.M. In addition to the usual household chores, the daytime worker took the elderly woman out of the house several times a week. She would take her for a ride, a walk, or shopping. She also was able to convince the widow to attend a neighborhood senior center that provided transportation for her visits at least once a week.

Another very sweet elderly lady who lived alone in her apartment was very lonely and wanted some companionship. She was depressed and needed reassurance. The Outreach aide provided her with someone to talk to and was regarded as a friend.

-✖-

A very energetic and outgoing seventy-eight-year-old woman lived in a small house in a rural town. Her home had a living-dining room, kitchen, and powder room on the first floor, and two bedrooms and a bath on the second floor. Although she was born in a city she has spent the last 50 years in this rural area. When she was a teenager she joined an order of nuns, and became an elementary teacher in a religious school. After five years she left the nuns and through the advice of a close older friend she attended a beautician school. Upon completion of the course she was placed in a beauty parlor in the vicinity of her present home.

This woman, Diane Harris, met her husband while working on this job. After she got married, Diane opened her own beauty parlor in her home. She has three children, two boys and a girl. She is extremely proud of her three children and their families and spoke glowingly of their many accomplishments. Both sons live quite far away, but she visits the one who lives on the West coast at least once a year. The other son lives much closer and has a summer house in Diane's area.

Her daughter, who is divorced, now lives with her and operates the beauty parlor. This daughter was divorced at about the time when Diane was ready to retire. Therefore Diane gave her daughter the beauty parlor, since she had previously been trained and worked as a beautician. Diane still assists in the shop occasionally.

Although Diane appears to be in relatively good health, thirty-five years ago she was severely ill with bleeding ulcers. "I was at death's door and had to have an operation," she said. "But I'm as good as new now."

Diane is a youthful-looking, tall, slim woman who speaks in a somewhat gruff voice. After her retirement she looked for some part-time work. "I had to do something. I have been so active all of my life," she explained. She was hired as director of community services in her village. This job was funded under the Green Thumb program, by the federal government. She was paid for twenty hours' work a week, but, as she commented, there were many times when she put in additional hours. She apparently loved the work and was extremely creative in developing programs and activities for the middle-aged and older people in her community and the surrounding area.

Diane took groups on a regular basis to a YMCA for exercise and swimming programs. She arranged for transportation from a retired man who owned a fifteen-passenger van and was delighted to drive them to and from their various activities. When her special trips to the theater and other outings involved more people, she hired a charter bus and charged a small fee to cover the cost. She also arranged trips to the urban shopping malls where the people could spend the day browsing and having lunch.

Since the area where Diane lives is too small to support a senior center, she started an informal social club that meets weekly at her house and serves a similar purpose. This club has about twenty-five members, ranging in age from fifty to eighty-two. They meet every Thursday afternoon right after lunch for three or four hours. Diane is the coordinator and she opens each meeting with a brief overview of scheduled activities and trips for the coming weeks. She also discusses any pertinent local, county, or state legislation that the members should know about. She will occasionally describe a book or article that she thinks would interest the women.

After the more formal part of the meeting, coffee, tea, and cake are served. Each week a different member supplies the refreshments. Each member contributes twenty-five cents a week to cover the cost of the paper goods and incidentals. There is a great deal of social interaction and people have formed close friendships in this club. They obviously care for each other and offer a great deal of mutual aid and support. The club is involved in various fund-raising drives, such as bake sales and small craft fairs. The money is used to subsidize the group's outings for those who cannot pay the full amount. The latter half of the meeting is usually devoted to some handiwork, such as crocheting, knitting, or quilting.

The club sponsors picnics and covered dish and pot-luck suppers to which the rest of the community is invited. Diane has also arranged for seminars on health and nutrition. There have been speakers on a variety of topics, and annual blood pressure screenings. A lawyer from a nearby community donated his services for six years, giving legal advice and writing wills at no cost. According to Diane, if not for this social club and its activities, its members would "not do anything."

Diane gave up her job recently, since she claimed that she did not want to be tied down to working a set amount of time each week. However, she still runs the social club and still arranges two or three overnight trips a year. She seems to be working almost as hard now without receiving a salary.

Legal Services

Legal service is sometimes available to the elderly. In some communities only low-income people are eligible, but those with higher incomes can get some initial help or at least a referral to a reputable lawyer. Legal services handle many types of civil matters including wills, public benefits, housing, utility bills, evictions, security deposits, consumer contracts, and family problems.

A seventy-six-year-old widow named Doris has lived all her married life in the downstairs unit of a duplex house, which she and her husband bought fifty years ago. She has been widowed for fifteen years. Doris has had emotional problems—the death of her husband aggravated this condition. During this grieving period, her brother-in-law asked her to sign over her house to him, promising that he would take care of it and allow her to stay in the house rent-free for the rest of her life. Since Doris was not coping very well at that time, she agreed, but did not get anything in writing from her brother-in-law.

A few years later, her brother-in-law tried to evict her. Doris contacted a local social agency for help and they referred her to the county legal services. This agency took her brother-in-law to court and Doris won the case: the judge ruled that she must be allowed to remain in the house for the rest of her life. This was a very important ruling for Doris. With her fragile emotional state, she could have landed in an institution if she had been forced to move. She needed the stable environment of her own home in order to continue to function.

Peter, a seventy-eight-year-old widower, had lived in a one-bedroom apartment for twenty years. The landlord decided to convert the apartment house to a condominium. Under state law, elderly renters were granted a protected tenancy status: they had the right to continue as renters for forty years after a condominium conversion. Despite this law, the landlord tried to evict Peter, claiming that he had failed to file the necessary papers with the municipality. However, Peter told the legal services lawyer that he had sent these papers to the landlord and the landlord was supposed to forward these to the local clerk. The lawyer won the case and Peter was given protected tenancy rights and allowed to continue to rent his apartment.

Another condominium protected tenancy case concerned Bertha, an elderly widow. She was living in a rent-controlled unit in a garden apartment complex. When this building went condominium, Bertha was granted protected tenancy and allowed to continue to live in the complex as a renter. A few months later a fire in the complex severely damaged eight apartments, including Bertha's. She lost all her furnishings and belongings in the fire. Bertha found a temporary apartment at twice the rent she had been paying. She really could not afford it, but couldn't find anything cheaper in the neighborhood she knew.

Two months later, the landlord sent her a letter that terminated her lease and refunded her security deposit. She was devastated since she had lived in that apartment complex for many years and had many close friends and neighbors. Bertha wrote to the governor for help. His office referred her letter to the state agency on aging which then contacted the legal services agency in her area. The lawyers were able to prove that the eviction was illegal because the landlord did not have the right to terminate the protected tenancy agreement. The court ruled that the landlord either had to restore her apartment or give her an equivalent one.

Larry, a single seventy year old, lived in an apartment in a high-rise building. He was very hard of hearing and played his radio and TV at high volume. His neighbors complained to the landlord about the excessive noise. After many failed attempts to get Larry to turn down the volume, the landlord finally served him with an eviction notice. When legal services got this case, they immediately referred Larry to a social agency for help with his hearing loss. He was given a hearing test and fitted with a hearing aid. With his new device, Larry was able to reduce the volume on his radio and TV. The judge overturned the eviction on condition that Larry use his hearing aid and reduce the noise level in his apartment. The landlord and the neighbors were pleased with this decision.

An elderly couple who owned their own home had cosigned their grandchildren's car loan applications. These older people did not understand what cosigning meant and mistakenly assumed that they bore no responsibility for the loans. When their grandchildren defaulted on these loans, the auto dealers sued the couple. Since the only asset the couple had was their home, they would have been forced to sell the house in order to pay off the loans. Here again, legal services was able to come to the rescue. After hearing the case, the court worked out a compromise that was acceptable to both parties. The couple could remain in their own home but a lien was placed against the house for the amount of the loan. The payment would not have to be made until the couple died or sold the house. The car dealers were also directed to try collecting payment from the actual car owners.

Another type of service that the legal services agencies can offer is to help frail but mentally competent elderly to draw up "durable powers of attorney." This document enables a family member, or any other person that the senior designates, to act as his or her agent in case of disability that interferes with the ability to carry out usual fiscal responsibilities. The agent can pay bills, balance the checking account, cash checks, file tax returns, and act as a representative in any court. However, this power can be exercised only when the older person is no longer capable of taking care of these matters himself or herself.

Transportation Services

Transportation is another service that is available in some form in most areas. Many states offer reduced fares for the elderly on trains and buses; in some parts of the country older people can ride public vehicles free. Some localities have free vans for senior citizens that run on a regular route to shopping areas. Others offer "dial-a-ride" service in which an elderly person can call a day in advance and arrange to be picked up and returned home again for doctor or hospital visits. A large urban area has a program called Easy Rider which has vans for transporting elderly who are unable to use public transportation. The user must schedule this ride in advance and priority is given for medical appointments. There is a nominal charge for this service.

In a large city in the Northeast the elderly living in a cooperative apartment development had to travel twenty blocks to the nearest supermarket. Since this was too far for them to walk to and return with heavy groceries, they needed some form of transportation. A few of the more resourceful people visited the neighborhood police station and told the captain of their plight. He assigned a police van that was free part of the week to take them shopping two times a week. The driver also helped them unload their groceries and carried them to the elevator. This made life much easier for these tenants.

In most rural areas of West Virginia, an arrangement has been made with local grocery stores to deliver groceries to homebound older people. This service is free to seniors who cannot get to the store and shop on their own. Area senior centers sponsor this service and pay mileage costs to the participating stores. The centers solicit donations from their communities to help defray the costs.[1]

Food Services

The Nutrition Program is federally funded and has sites throughout the United States. It offers a hot noon meal five days a week in a congregate setting to low- and moderate-income elderly and others who cannot prepare their own hot meals. The meal is free but a small donation is asked of those who can afford it. Almost all the sites provide transportation. The seniors usually arrive a little before lunch and some will stay an hour or so later to socialize or play cards. This program is housed in YMCAs and YWCAs, senior citizen projects, senior centers, and other types of community buildings.

I visited two nutrition sites in upstate New York. They had both been in existence since the program started about fifteen years ago. One was located in a firehouse and had a very large airy dining room. There were about thirty people in attendance sitting at four tables. They were chatting away and appeared to be having a good time. The group was composed of almost an equal number of men and women. Some of the men said that they had been coming to this lunch for seven years.

Most of the attendees were eager to discuss how they felt about this program. One man said, "I'm single. I get a darn good meal and I don't have to cook."

Another offered, "The cooking is good and it only costs $1.50. I get good food and good companionship."

A single woman said, "I meet very good friends here and I love to hear the gossip."

"It's something to do. It breaks up the day."

"I found out where I could get a cheap dentist and learn all sorts of other things from my friends here."

"It's cheaper than eating at home and I don't like to cook. I like to meet everyone and have somebody to talk to."

A legally blind woman told me, "I live alone and come for the company. It's good to get together and have somebody to talk to."

In general the feeling of most of the older people was that this was an important daily activity for them since it gave them a well-balanced, nutritious meal and an opportunity to meet and talk with a number of different people each day. As one woman put it, "It gets you out in circulation." The nutrition program helped replace the friends who had died or moved away. It also offered the opportunity for volunteering in setting up, serving, and clearing the tables for those elderly who wanted to be of service.

Helen Stout, a ninety-one-year-old widow, has been coming to the meals program for many years. She has lived in her present house since 1947. She has three children, two sons and a daughter, who all live in the city about a two-hour drive away. She is very close to her family and they visit quite frequently. She is a very independent person with a delicious sense of humor and a very upbeat personality.

She is in relatively good health for a woman of her age but recently has become hard of hearing. She worked for many years as a nurse. When she retired she continued to give service to her community by going to the local hospital on a weekly basis and mending bed linens and patients' clothes. She had to stop when it became too difficult for her to run the electric sewing machine. The nutrition program gave her an easier volunteer activity and she has enjoyed helping to set the tables. Helen is determined to stay in her own home. She confessed that she still has an attic full of her husband's and children's things which she treasures. She is an avid reader, does her own housework, and walks four miles at least two or three times a week.

Senior Centers

Many senior centers serve breakfast and lunch and some participate in the federal nutrition program. This type of facility usually offers a comprehensive package of services and activities and is open for a full day. In some communities the senior center functions as the major resource for all the elderly in that locality.

Sally Davis, a long-time widow who was eighty-seven years old, had become very depressed, had stopped eating, and spent most of the day in bed. She had been an unusually outgoing and active person who was very involved in community organizations. Her daughter lived about an hour away but she drove to her mother's house three mornings a week to get her dressed and give her breakfast. Sally's eyesight had begun to deteriorate badly and her daughter-in-law had been critically ill—these two conditions seem to have caused her depression. Since getting out of the house improves her emotional state, the daughter has encouraged Sally to attend the senior center.

The senior center has made a big difference in Sally's mental outlook on life. She has found some friends at the center who care about her and she takes pleasure in being a helper. She thoroughly enjoyed participating in a fashion show. The center staff always make sure that she goes on all their trips and call her in advance to remind her.

Her center is open seven days a week and serves breakfast. There is a nutrition site four blocks away, but for those elderly who prefer to eat their noon meal at the center tea, coffee, rolls and butter, and snacks are always available. The staff feels that having food available all day encourages older people to attend and helps to make them feel welcome. On weekends, the center shows feature films, runs bingo games, and serves lunch or a substantial snack. Transportation is also provided on weekends.

The center averages between 75 and 125 participants during the week and attracts at least 100 on weekends. Like many other such facilities, it functions as a multipurpose center with social events, crafts, a speaker's program, parties, and other entertainment. It also offers a dial-a-ride service to and from doctors, dentists, hospitals, and social agencies in town and in neighboring communities, and runs a minibus for shopping and other errands.

In addition to all the social programs and transportation services, this center offers a wide range of other services, including information and referral, Outreach, bookmobile, Mr. Fixit, notary, hypertension screening, tax assistance, and exercise programs.

Another senior center I visited had a few rather unusual activities. One was an intergenerational program in which high school students taught older people about computers so that they could communicate better with their grandchildren. It also offered courses in comparative religion and about antiques.

According to one senior center director, a center serves as a focal point for the elderly and provides access to services in a nonthreatening manner. "It keeps their support system alive and well, and in a positive way it fills the voids caused by the many losses they experience. Best of all, a senior center helps older people remain independent and in control of their lives."

The National Institute of Senior Centers (NISC) is in the process of developing an accreditation program that will establish national standards. These will be flexible and will reflect both the community and the elderly population it serves.

A lively and outgoing woman of eighty-one named Rita Thomas was most eager to tell me how the senior center she had been attending for the past eleven years had changed her life. Rita was born in Europe and came to the United States when she was eighteen. She married an American reporter. They had two sons, one a successful businessman and the other a college professor. She is very proud of their achievements. After twenty-two years of marriage Rita divorced her husband. Two years later Rita remarried, this time to a farmer in New Jersey. She found this environment too confining and after 11 years divorced her second husband. She has been single ever since and enjoys her freedom and privacy.

Rita moved back to the city and found an attractive one-bedroom apartment in the center of town. When she first arrived in this country she did not know any English and therefore had to work as a seamstress in a factory. She later worked as a masseuse and a beautician. After she learned the language she found work in a social agency and became a supervisor of the clerical staff. She held this job until retirement at age sixty-nine.

Rita found herself at loose ends after retirement. Some of her friends had moved away, others had died. She was beginning to feel lonely and in need of some structured activity. Eleven years ago, she discovered a large and active senior center not far from where she lived and she has been an extremely involved participant ever since.

The center introduced her to many new activities and hobbies and helped her form new friendships. "The center gave me an extended family," she said, "and my life began to take a happy shape. I didn't feel alone and isolated anymore." But, she confessed, "I got so involved that I found I had no time for myself and so I've had to drop some activities."

Rita does take advantage of most of the programs offered at the center and she is also one of the twelve members on the board of directors. Over the years, she has taken classes in art, ceramics, playing the recorder, folk dancing, ballroom dancing, knitting, arts and crafts, and bridge. She participates in discussion groups and legislative action. She has recently joined a writing class that has stimulated her to write short autobiographical stories. Rita has taken on the responsibility of scheduling and managing trips to Atlantic City, which she thoroughly enjoys. She volunteers her services and administers medication to those people at the center who require it. She also acts as a counselor and says, "I love it. I just love it. I'm very good with people that have problems."

The center offers its members free tickets to the theater and the opera, and Rita takes advantage of the service. She also takes occasional weekend trips and has been spending a month in Mexico each of the past few winters. She kept reiterating how much the center means to her and what a difference it has made in her life. "I get a great deal and I give a great deal. We all get older, but I get younger," she exclaimed. The most unexpected result of Rita's center activities has been meeting Robert Stone; Rita and Robert are the same age, have become fast friends, and go everywhere together.

Robert Stone was a thoughtful and articulate person who shared Rita's enthusiasm for the senior center. He had been married for thirty-four years and had had a very happy marriage. He has two children, a son and a daughter, and they each live about a half an hour away. When he was first married during the Great Depression, they were fortunate to find an apartment in public housing. He earned a marginal living as a taxi driver, but during the war he worked in a defense plant as an aircraft mechanic. During those years he was able to save enough money to buy a taxi medallion and his own taxicab after the war. His business prospered so that he could afford to buy a moderate-income cooperative apartment, and to send his children to college.

Robert is a very intelligent person who had hoped to be a mechanical engineer. However, his mother was a widow and after he had finished high school he was forced to go to work to help support the family. He said, "Since I couldn't build bridges I thought I could try to build an organization." He became involved in developing an association of individual taxicab owners. He took an active role in the association which started with fifty members and grew to have over two hundred. He organized their radio-call system and acted as the chief troubleshooter.

About 11 years ago Robert's wife died and he was quite devastated. He moved in with his daughter temporarily since he needed close family support. He said that his daughter "kept pushing single women at me, but they weren't for me. So I decided to move back home and find a congenial social setting for myself." He also felt that his four-and-a-half-room apartment was too large, so he exchanged it for a three-room apartment in the same development.

He was told that the senior center was a good place to meet new people. When he first saw it, he was not favorably impressed because "the people looked so old and decrepit." However, when he saw the schedule of activities for the month he felt it was worth "giving it a try." After a few days at the center he was completely sold on its program and has been attending on a regular basis ever since.

Robert is as involved in the center as Rita is, although in his own areas of interest. He serves on the executive board and attends every meeting. When one of the instructors learned that he was mechanically inclined, he asked Robert to run the movie projector, which he now does once a month. He became interested in the drama group which meets once a week and he took courses at the center in acting and playwriting. Now he writes skits and one-act plays, mainly adaptations of stories he has read. His skits and plays are produced at the center about four times a year and have received high praise. He is an avid reader and says, "All my new activities here have helped improve my vocabulary and opened up my communicative abilities. From a taxi driver I have become an intellectual."

Robert feels that finding Rita was one of the nicest things that has happened to him at the center. Although he has found many new acquaintances she is his only real friend. Rita makes friends quickly and easily. Robert says, "I need an outgoing person and Rita is very much like my wife in personality. I'm laid back in a new social situation and am very cautious when I first meet people."

Both Robert and Rita are very enthusiastic about the senior center and feel that it has greatly enriched their lives. However, Robert was the more introspective and analytical of the two and was eager to share with me the reasons why he thought people attended this center. He felt that the basic reason was loneliness, but he also believed that participants appreciated the savings in terms of the free or very inexpensive lunches, free theater tickets, and low-cost day and overnight trips. The many programs and opportunities for volunteer activities were important benefits that could not be obtained elsewhere. Robert added that the center also allowed those people who did not want to be active to have a place where they could sit and read (the center had an extensive library), and engage in passive recreation in a social setting.

A typical week's programs at this urban senior center consist of ceramics, memory class, chair exercise, Spanish conversation, social line dancing and games, drawing and painting, sewing, social action, drama, recycling crafts, bridge, exercise-dancing, crafts, piano and song, knitting and crocheting, hair care, discussion, chorus, folk dance, and bingo. Special programs for a typical month included films, a membership meeting, a lecture on local history, a play, and a birthday party.

For many older people who live alone, the hours spent at a senior center or a nutrition site constitute the focal point of each day, and the meal served may be the main source of nutrition. Meals-on-Wheels programs are often operated out of these centers; volunteers deliver a hot lunch and cold food for the evening meal, once a day, for the housebound elderly.

Home Aides

Agencies can supply homemakers to help the elderly with cleaning, laundry, cooking, shopping, and personal needs like bathing and dressing. Many of these same agencies provide home health-care personnel. Regular home visits by registered nurses, licensed practical nurses, nursing assistants, home health aides, or therapists are usually obtained on the recommendation of a physician, often through a hospital social-service unit.

Fees vary, depending upon the agency and the services provided. Some costs may be eligible for reimbursement by Medicare and private health insurance. All persons sixty-five and over are eligible for Medicare, the government insurance program that pays part of the elderly's medical and hospital costs through Social Security. Medicare will pay for skilled nursing care, but only after a hospital stay and only for three months. Neither Medicare nor most private insurers will cover the cost of long-term home health care or custodial nursing home care.[2]

Adult Day Care

Adult day care is available for the less mentally competent, the physically handicapped, or the socially deprived elderly. These programs usually operate five days a week for a full day and offer both medical and social supportive services. They provide meals and transportation. Many of these day-care centers are subsidized by nonprofit agencies; the services at subsidized centers are free or cost a minimal amount. Private adult day-care agencies charge a daily fee.

A typical day-care center in an urban area offers both medical and social day-care services including recreation, hot meals, transportation, counseling, health screening, supervision of medications, treatments as prescribed by the doctor, physical, speech, and occupational therapies, family education and support, and assessment and case management.[3]

One such day-care center I visited is housed in its own building and is sponsored by a nonprofit religious organization. It has an enrollment of seventy-seven people and an average daily attendance of forty-five. It is an attractive facility with one very large community room, a number of smaller crafts and card rooms, and a kitchen. The spaces are bright and cheerful and the place is humming with activity. At large and small tables throughout the center groups of people were sitting and talking. Some were playing dominoes and other games, some reading, some doing crafts, some painting. The groups looked animated and appeared to be having a good time.

This center is open five days a week from 8 A.M. to 4 P.M. and serves breakfast, lunch, and snacks. A flexible schedule enables those who prefer it to come later in the morning or to attend just two or three days a week. In addition to the medical services available at the center, people needing special rehabilitation and physiotherapy are transported to a nearby hospital. A few times a year special trips and picnics are scheduled. When the weather permits, the participants are taken to a park where they can walk or just sit and contemplate nature. Special events and parties are scheduled for holidays. Elementary and high school students visit from time to time and interact with the elderly. At Halloween, they come dressed in costumes and play games with the participants at the center. When I was at the center, four young children came with their teacher and visited with some of the older people.

This center is free for low-income elderly. For those who can afford it, the fee is $30 a day, including transportation. Participants range in age from fifty-five to ninety-two.

Sybil, an eighty-two-year-old widow, has been coming to the center for over a year. She has been widowed for more than forty years. She had one son, but he died. She has a younger sister who lives on the West coast and a niece and nephew who live close by. Sybil lives alone in a small two-story townhouse, with a large living-dining area and kitchen on the first floor and one bedroom and bath upstairs. She had been a factory worker and a nurse's aide when she was younger but once she was married she stayed at home and was a housewife.

Sybil is an outgoing and attractive person who led a quiet life and occupied herself with friends and church activities. Two years ago she had a stroke that left her with a weakness on her left side. She is now in a wheelchair but can walk a few steps if she is aided. She is able to manage at home because her nephew converted the downstairs room into a bedroom so that she would not have to be carried up and down stairs.

After she had recovered from her stroke, she wanted to remain living in her own home. Her nephew felt that this would not be possible unless she attended an adult day-care center on a regular basis. Sybil said that when it was explained to her, "it sounded like an old folk's home and I wouldn't have any of that." She resisted until the center director visited her a few times and encouraged her to come to the center for a few days on a trial basis. After about a week, Sybil decided that she really liked it and has been a regular participant ever since.

Sybil is an unusually friendly person and has made many friends. "We get along real good," she said. "I just enjoy myself. Something is always going on. And talking to people all the time makes me very happy." In addition to visiting with her friends at the center, she enjoys the classes in writing and drawing, the poetry recitals, the group singing, and the twice-a-week church services where they sing hymns. She also participates in the kitchen activities in the afternoons when a small group prepares vegetables and other food for the next day's meals.

At home, Sybil manages with the help of a home health aide during the week and a neighbor who comes for an hour or so on the weekends. Her niece and nephew do the weekly shopping and visit with her when they can. They are very fond of her. However, if not for the day-care center, Sybil would undoubtedly have had to go to a nursing home.

-✳-

Maude Sidney has been attending the day-care center ever since it opened. She is seventy-five years old and has been divorced for many years. Her husband was in the navy and she traveled with him all over the country. Since her divorce she has lived in a two-story attached house, with living room, dining room, and kitchen on the first floor and three bedrooms and bath upstairs. She was born in the South but moved to the Northeast forty-five years ago. She had no children of her own but she raised her sister's daughter and granddaughter as if they were her own.

She is a tall well-built woman. A high school graduate, she worked for the railroad as a blue-collar worker. She retired fifteen years ago but missed the comraderie of her fellow workers. Although she is in relatively good health (she had cataracts removed from both eyes and takes medication for hypertension), she needs the day-care program for socialization. She attends only three times a week; she bowls with a team one day each week and she volunteers at her church another day.

Her life at the center has settled into a pleasant routine. She likes the arts and crafts and sewing. "I like to work with my hands," she explained, "and I have been making flower pot hangers and am now working with clay." She also plays bingo and dominoes. Maude is not particularly outgoing but wants to have people around her even if she is just reading. She brings her own newspaper and often will spend part of the morning reading articles to one of the men who is blind. When I asked her how many friends she had at the center, she replied, "I consider them all my friends." She also added, "I like the center. I miss the people here if I have to be home sick."

-✳-

For one couple in their mid-eighties the adult day-care center saved their marriage and prevented the wife from having to go to a nursing home. Phyllis and Mark had been married for over sixty years and had been living in their present house for fifty of those years. Mark had been a successful businessman who has become rather cantankerous since his retirement. Phyllis had stayed home and raised her family. They have three daughters who all live out-of state but are caring and try to offer as much support as their parents will allow.

About two years ago Phyllis fell and broke her hip. She was hospitalized and then sent home with an aide for help. This fall was most traumatic and she became bitter and angry. Her emotional state made living with her very difficult for her husband who could not cope with her moods. The situation came to a head when his wife had to return to the hospital because of a serious bladder infection that caused her to be incontinent. The hospital referred her to a rehabilitation center since she was refusing to walk or to help herself get well.

The social worker at the center felt that she needed a day-care program to continue making progress in both her emotional and physical conditions. Phyllis is now attending a medical day-care center three times a week. She participates in all the programs, has made some new friends, and her attitude toward life has improved greatly. She is now walking with a cane and her emotional health has changed markedly. Her new attitude has also had a positive effect on her husband's attitude and their marriage. The daughters are relieved and find that they can be of more help now since there is much less anger and recrimination in their parents' household.

Adult day-care centers serve the frail elderly and help them maintain or restore their maximal functional abilities. A growing need for this type of facility seems to be matched by the rapid growth of these programs. In 1978, there were 300 adult day-care centers in the country in 40 states, serving over 5,000 people. Today 2,000 centers in all the states serve over 70,000 elderly people.[4]

Volunteering and Employment Opportunities

In addition to all the services available to older people, most communities offer volunteer and employment opportunities as well. ACTION, a federal agency, administers several volunteer programs through local grantees; among them are the Foster Grandparent Program (FGP), Senior Companion Program (SCP), and Retired Senior Volunteer Program (RSVP). The first two, FGP and SCP, offer low-income people age sixty and over the chance to work twenty hours a week for a small stipend, with expenses paid and the added benefit of an annual physical exam. Trained and supervised by sponsoring agencies (schools, hospitals, day-care centers) foster grandparents serve four hours per day tending the needs of mentally and physically handicapped children. Volunteers in the SCP assist homebound, chronically disabled elderly; indeed, delivery of many in-home services depends on these older volunteers.

RSVP, with no income limits, serves a variety of organizations. Volunteer stations may include courts, schools, libraries, day-care centers, hospitals, Boy Scout and Girl Scout offices, economic-development agencies, and other community service centers. Volunteers are not paid, but they may be reimbursed for transportation, meals, and other out-of-pocket expenses connected with their service. They receive a brief orientation from the local RSVP project director and in-service instruction after placement.

The retired executive who misses his old business milieu may be able to continue to participate through SCORE, Service Corps of Retired Executives, or ACE, Active Corps of Executives. These programs of the U.S. Small Business Administration link seasoned volunteer businesspeople with owners and managers of small local businesses who seek management or technical counseling. Volunteers provide their expertise for free, but they do receive reimbursement for their transportation and other expenses.

For some elderly people, earning money may be a more urgent matter than keeping busy or being of service. But finding a job is difficult for most older people. To help provide employment opportunities for low-income people who are fifty-five or older, the U.S. Department of Labor subsidizes community service projects administered by public or nonprofit agencies or organizations. Projects must contribute to the general welfare of communities as well as increase the number of employment opportunities for older people. Some national contractors approved for funding are Green Thumb (an affiliate of the National Farmers Union), American Association of Retired Persons (AARP), National Council on the Aging (NCOA), and the U.S. Forestry Service. NCOA, for example, provides work and training opportunities for approximately ten thousand older persons each year.[5]

Educational and Recreational Opportunities

Many older people want the opportunity to continue or to brush up on their education. Others want the intellectual stimulation that learning provides. Most colleges offer continuing education courses or allow the elderly to audit courses on a space-available basis. Many of these courses are free or are offered for a minimal fee.

The Elderhostel organization offers courses throughout the United States and in many foreign countries. Courses usually run for one week; the fee for the course includes tuition and room and board. Janet and Richard, both widowed and in their early seventies, actually met at an Elderhostel week. They not only enjoyed their courses but fell in love and were married. They continue to attend Elderhostel courses at least once or twice a year; they believe that Elderhostel not only provides stimulating vacations but also allows them to visit different parts of the country and make new friends.

Since they both were college graduates and had worked as professionals before they retired, they were interested in expanding their fields of knowledge and have been attending a local college two days a week. They each take different courses and spend the better part of the day at the school. They bring lunch; after their morning classes they meet together with other students in the lunchroom. They enjoy this social hour where they can exchange ideas and information from their morning classes. As Janet says with a great deal of enthusiasm, "I find the classes so stimulating. It keeps us young. Keeps us growing. It makes us feel alive." In the afternoon, they will often attend an interesting special lecture.

In addition to these educational opportunities, there are classes at senior and community centers, and at local high schools. In some parts of the country, such as New York City and Florida, groups of retired professionals have formed teaching cooperatives, where the teachers donate their services and the elderly students pay only a modest fee to cover the administrative costs (see chapter 8).

Recreational opportunities are available to the elderly in senior and community centers, schools, and senior clubs. In addition, the federal government issues passes to all national parks, monuments, historic sites, and recreation areas that charge entrance fees. These passes are called Golden Age Passports and are available to anyone sixty-two years of age or older. Most states also offer free admission for senior citizens to the state parks.

A Helping Hand

State and Area Agencies on Aging and Other Community Resources

I have just been exploring some of the services and opportunities available to older people. How does one find out about these services and where do they exist in the community? There are many resources that can be of help but the best place to start is the area agency on aging or the state unit on aging.

All area agencies and most state agencies on aging have information and referral services. Many have a toll-free hot line specifically for this purpose. Staff are available during regular business hours, and there is usually provision for leaving a recorded message at other times. Written requests for information are answered very promptly. I visited one state and two area agencies on aging and followed the information and referral specialists' activities on several different days.

State Aging Hot Line

During a typical month, the state agency receives over four thousand requests for help on the hot line. These range from questions on boarding care facilities to weatherization assistance. The largest number of requests are for information concerning program materials and entitlements. Other frequent inquiries are about life-line and pharmaceutical materials, Medicare, housing, and caregiver assistance.

The state's hot line carefully trains and supervises its information and referral staff. They appear to be caring and sensitive people who handle the telephone calls with a great deal of patience and skill. They try to evaluate the older persons they talk with in terms of their frailty and ability to follow through. After the caller is given the name and telephone number of the appropriate agency, he or she is advised to recontact the hot line if he or she is not satisfied with the referral or needs further help. Some of the elderly who call are just lonely and want someone to talk to; they are usually referred to a telephone reassurance service, a friendly visiting service, or a senior center.

Very often the caller is not an older person but a younger family member, a daughter or son. A daughter contacted the hot line about her eighty-two-year-old mother who was living in a two-bedroom apartment about ten miles away from her. She thought her mother was in fairly good physical health, but she was becoming concerned because she had noticed little lapses of memory and slight changes in her mother's behavior. On several occasions the gas stove has been left on, and the refrigerator door left ajar.

The mother eats alone and complains that she is lonely. Her daughter is not sure what her mother is eating and whether she is getting the proper nutrition. However, her parent wants to remain in her own home and does not want to move in with her daughter. The mother has a modest income and her daughter has tried to get her to accept a live-in companion but so far has not been successful in obtaining one. The hot-line specialist suggested that the mother see a physician to check if there was any medical problem causing the memory lapses and behavior changes, and referred the daughter to the Title 5 employment resource specialist in her area for a possible companion. The staff member also recommended that the daughter contact her area agency on aging information and referral specialist if she needed any further help.

A husband of sixty-five and a wife of seventy-two had lived in a very protected semi-institutional setting for most of their married life. They now lived in a small apartment and did not know how to manage their limited income or how to structure their day. They tended to spend their time at shopping centers and eating at restaurants. These pursuits were unsatisfactory, not to say expensive The hotline referred them to a nearby senior center that had a meals program, activities, and an outreach service. The couple was able to get their breakfast and main meal (lunch) at the center, so they did not have to spend money at restaurants. They enjoyed the games and socialization and found some new friends. In addition, the outreach worker was able to gain their confidence and connected them with other government programs that they were entitled to, programs that helped them to manage better on their small income.

A widow of sixty-seven had lost her husband two years ago. Her mortgage was $517 a month, and her total income from her husband's Social Security and her part-time job was $800. She needed additional income and was also somewhat lonely. The state information and referral specialist suggested sharing her home with another single older woman and referred her to the state housing office for a list of home-share agencies. She was also referred to the county match agency for specific help in finding a suitable housemate.

A sixty-year-old widow lived in her own home. She had severely ulcerated legs and could not stand for any period of time. A direct referral was made to the area agency on aging. They arranged for transportation for flu shots and other medical appointments. Since she was unable to food shop, had difficulty cooking, and was essentially homebound, she was eligible for the Meals-on-Wheels program. This widow had been unaware of the area agency and of the services it provided, and was most grateful for the referral from the state division on aging.

A man and his seventy-eight-year-old mother lived in their own home. The son worked and was able to pay for services for his parent but did not know how to obtain them. His mother had a chronic inner ear problem that caused difficulty with her equilibrium and she needed someone to houseclean and prepare her lunch. The son was referred to the area agency on aging. They arranged for the mother to have a homemaker come to the house for a few hours a day, five days a week. This program has a sliding fee scale so that the son was able to pay for these necessary services.

An elderly woman who lived alone in her own home did not drive and was unable to get to the nearest food market. She was fortunate to have a neighbor who had a car and did her shopping for her. When he died, she was devastated and did not know where to turn for help. The state hot line was able to refer her to the local senior center which had a van that took older people to the supermarket twice a week. This service solved her problem and relieved her of having to rely on neighbors or other people for shopping.

A seventy-two-year-old widow who lived in her own home had a furnace in need of repair. She had no heat and called public service for emergency help. Unfortunately, she could not afford the cost of the repair and did not know what to do. She called the state hot line, and they in turn referred her to her area agency on aging. This agency determined that she was eligible for the weatherization program. Her furnace was repaired immediately and at no cost to her.

The state information and referral service was contacted by a sixty-seven-year-old widow who was lonely and wanted some daily contact with people. She was referred to the area agency on aging for help. An outreach worker was sent to her home and found out that she was under a doctor's care. The woman gave her permission to call him and the outreach worker learned that the woman was suffering from an anxiety neurosis and needed some companionship and reassurance. Arrangements were made to connect her with telephone reassurance and friendly visiting programs, and the outreach worker kept in weekly contact with her thereafter.

In addition to the many calls received by the state aging hot line and information and referral specialists for assistance by older people and their families, the agencies receive requests for help by mail either directly or through the governor's office. They are usually able to satisfy these requests by sending information on specific state or federal programs and/or giving referrals to the local area agency on aging.

The written replies explain the function of the area agency and also indicate that the state office may be able to supply further information which can be obtained by calling the hot-line number, free of charge.

A son wrote to the governor and asked for help with a zoning problem. This letter was forwarded to the state agency on aging for a reply. It seems that the son had been recently married and had decided to convert the upstairs of his mother's home into an apartment for his new wife and himself. He felt that the new arrangement would be best for his mother and would enable her to continue to live independently. After doing some construction, he discovered that the zoning laws did not permit him to install a second kitchen. His only alternative was to apply to the municipality for a variance. The son was asking if the state could offer any help in this situation.

He was advised that zoning was a local responsibility—the state could not intervene. However, he was referred to the state housing agency who might be able to offer some specific suggestions on his presentation before the zoning board. Two American Association of Retired Persons (AARP) publications were sent to him, *A Consumer's Guide to Accessory Apartments* and *Legal Issues in Accessory Apartments: Zoning and Covenants Restricting Land to Residential Uses.* He was also referred to the area agency on aging to see if the county's legal services could represent his mother at the zoning hearing.

The Division on Aging is also contacted by professionals writing on behalf of their clients. A very good example of this was a letter they received from a lawyer who represented a married couple. The husband was seventy-seven and the wife was seventy-five. The husband had had a recent heart bypass operation that had adversely affected the use of his right arm and right leg, and the wife suffered from diabetes, high blood pressure, and emphysema. The couple owned a mobile home but had no other assets. They had a total monthly income of $1,100. However, due to their health conditions they were having some financial problems. The lawyer was requesting literature on support services for which his clients would be eligible so that he could help them apply for them. He also wanted any information on financial assistance for their medical bills.

The division outlined the services offered on a county level and referred the lawyer to the area agency on aging's information and referral specialist for specific help with support services. The state agency enclosed two of their own publications, *Statewide Benefits for Older Persons* and *Federal Programs for Older Persons.* The latter specifically mentioned the Pharmaceutical Assistance to the Aged and Disabled program (PAAD), which enables a participant to pay only $2 for each prescription. A PAAD brochure was enclosed and the lawyer was advised to have his clients enroll in this program if they were eligible.

Area Agencies on Aging I & R

In many cases the state unit on aging information and referral (I & R) staff handles inquiries by referring the people to the area agency on aging for the specific help they require. I spent time at two such agencies in a northeastern state to find out about the kinds of problems they encountered and how they resolved them. One of these agencies received an average of 728 calls a month. Although the calls ranged from questions about health services to information about food stamps, the majority of the calls were concerned with transportation, housing, pharmaceutical assistance, doctors who made home visits, and the dental program.

A seventy-six-year-old-woman who lived alone in her own house was not paying her utility bills. Public Service called the area agency to tell them that they were going to have to cut off this woman's gas and electric due to nonpayment of her bills. The information and referral specialist asked that the service not be terminated until they could investigate the reason for nonpayment. Public Service agreed. The agency called the woman and told her that they were coming to see her about the gas and electricity. Since they did not know what they would find, they had staff from the city health and police departments accompany them.

They found a very fearful old lady who was very dirty and looked as if she had never changed her clothes. In addition, her house was filthy and very cluttered. It was apparent that she needed medical attention, so they took her to the hospital. The medical staff found that she was suffering from anemia and malnutrition. She was hospitalized for two weeks and then she was placed in a sheltered care home on a temporary basis for three more weeks. The area agency used the time to get her house fumigated and cleaned. They also visited her several times a week and brought her clean clothes. After she returned home, she was assigned a friendly visitor and some homemaking service.

Three sisters ranging in age from seventy-four to seventy-nine lived in an upstairs apartment in a two-family house. The unit had a kitchen, dining room, living room, bath, and two bedrooms. The youngest sister slept on a convertible bed in the living room. When the landlord raised the rent, the sisters called the area agency for help. The information and referral specialist determined that one of the sisters was eligible for SSI and PAAD, which improved their financial condition. In addition, they were given rental assistance (a Section 8 federal subsidy) which reduced their rent to only 30 percent of their income.

Another call came from an elderly man who required help with some medical problems. He needed a hearing aid and did not know where to obtain one he could afford. He was referred to a clinic that would test and fit him with a suitable aid and charge him according to a sliding scale. The clinic also provided follow-up service to make sure that the hearing aid was functioning properly. The caller also needed an eye doctor and a dentist. He was given the names of several in his neighborhood who take Medicare assignments.

A veteran who had lost his pension called. He was given the name and phone number of the person to contact at the Veterans of Foreign Wars Administration.

An elderly couple called and wanted to know how they could obtain safety locks on their front and back doors. They were given the phone number and name of the person to contact at the municipal police department for specific help with this problem. The police came to their home and evaluated their needs. In addition to installing locks, they secured the windows. These services were free.

The information and referral specialist gets many calls about the half-fare bus and train program. The office has the necessary forms and suggests that callers come to the office with their birth certificates, and the staff will help them fill out the forms. If they prefer, the forms with necessary instructions are mailed to the older people. In addition, the area agency is always available to help any elderly person fill out other forms, such as Medicare, medical insurance, life-line, and PAAD forms.

A widowed elderly woman who lived with her son in their own house had fallen and broken her wrist. Because she also had a bad heart she was hospitalized. She called the information and referral specialist upon her return home since she needed some home care during the day while her son worked. The office arranged for a homemaker to come in five days a week for four hours a day. The homemaker helps her get out of bed, gets her dressed, takes her for walks, tidies the house, and prepares her meals. Her son and daughter assist her on weekends. Also her neighbors are very supportive, and take turns visiting her on a regular basis after the homemaker leaves. When her son is away in the evening, the information and referral specialist, on her own time, visits her and helps her get ready for bed.

A very heavy widow 80 years of age lives in an apartment. She has bad eyesight and had a stroke which necessitates that she use a walker or the support of two canes. She is extremely independent and is determined to manage in her own home. She called the office on aging for help. They arranged for a homemaker who comes to the house six hours a day, five days a week. Since the widow has a modest income, she only pays part of the cost, $5 an hour. The information and referral specialist visited her and assisted her in filling out her PAAD and Medicare forms. Now, her neighbors check on her each evening.

The area agency on aging gets numerous calls for information on programs and services that the seniors hear about on the radio and TV or read about in the local newspapers. They are interested in learning the specific details, what the costs are, and how to apply. The staff are always available to answer their questions and/or to send them the appropriate brochures.

In many cases a younger relative calls the office on aging for help with a parent or other older person. A daughter who lived about six hundred miles away from her eighty-two-year-old mother called the agency because she felt that her mother could no longer manage to live alone. Although the daughter felt that the best solution would be for her mother to move in with her, her mother refused. The parent was a very frail old lady with beginning Alzheimer's disease.

The mother lived in a small one-bedroom apartment which was immaculate and beautifully furnished. An agency staff member visited the mother and found her to be an attractive, intelligent woman with some memory loss who was determined to continue to live in her apartment but was willing to accept any help to do this.

The area agency found a woman who lived in the same apartment building and was interested in a part-time job. After checking with the building manager as to her reliability and honesty, this neighbor was hired. She works five half days a week and makes breakfast, does the food shopping, cleans the apartment, and does the wash in the morning. She returns in the late afternoon and prepares and serves the older woman dinner. Until a senior companion can be found this neighbor has agreed to take her out and help relieve her loneliness. The elderly lady lives on the fourteenth floor and feels very isolated and alone. If not for the intervention of the area agency, this frail, somewhat disoriented woman would have to be cared for in a nursing home.

The other area agency on aging that I observed had an information and referral unit that functioned in a slightly different manner.

In addition to the usual answering of questions, referrals, and problem solving, they start each day with a Telephone Reassurance program. The staff, including some volunteers, spend from 8:30 to 10:00 each morning, checking, by phone, forty seniors who live alone and asked for this service. A typical recipient of the service is an eighty-three-year-old widow who lives alone and is homebound because of a broken hip. She wanted the service to allay her fears. She had fallen and had been found by the police unconscious on the floor. She did not want to repeat this scary experience. A woman in her early sixties with a history of heart problems asked for the service so that someone would check her health each day. When she suffered a heart attack and did not answer her phone, a rescue squad was sent immediately to her home. She was taken to the hospital, where she was treated and recovered.

The Telephone Reassurance program has a prearranged time so that each person in the program knows approximately the time he or she will be called. If there is no answer the first time the person is contacted, three more attempts are made before a close neighbor or the police are asked to go to the home. If the recipient of this service will be away during the call period, he or she must notify the program. An answering machine is checked each morning for messages before anyone is called.

Another service that is offered is a handyman-chore service. This is staffed entirely by community volunteers, ranging from college students to seniors. The service is free, but those who can afford it are asked to contribute the cost of the materials. This program not only helps with home maintenance and with minor repairs, but it also puts someone in the house who is trained to see if the older person is in need of any other services. The volunteers must meet as a group once a month but otherwise give as much or as little time as they wish.

An elderly woman in her early eighties lived in her own house. She was frail, with poor eyesight, emphysema, and a heart condition. She had requested help with raking leaves. However, when the volunteer worker arrived, he found the inside of the house was a mess and the outside in need of repair and maintenance. The food in the refrigerator was moldy, the sink was piled high with dirty dishes, and the entire house looked as if it had not been cleaned for a long time.

Six students from a local church washed the floors and the curtains, and scrubbed the entire house. The handyman volunteer assessed what needed to be repaired, and found leaky faucets, flaky ceilings, crumbling walls, and the entire inside and outside badly in need of painting. He did the minor repairs himself. Funds from the municipal block grant were used to hire professionals to fix the walls and ceilings. In addition, a homemaker was hired to do the cleaning and help with the cooking and shopping three times a week.

A ninety-year-old woman who lived in a two-story house was hard of hearing and had failing eyesight. She was having difficulty going up and down the stairs. She asked for a railing to help her navigate the steps.

An elderly couple needed help with the heavy housework and yardwork. A student was sent to wash the windows, take down and clean the curtains, and work in the yard. It also became apparent that they needed someone to clean the house on a regular basis. A high school student now comes in once a week and helps with the household chores.

In addition to the elderly themselves requesting this chore service, the area agency gets referrals from family, other agencies, hospitals, and doctors. This service was expanded about nine months ago to include a special clean-up day for any older person who requested it. This program has a roster of fifty-nine volunteers who give a total of approximately 182 hours a month. In a typical month thirty-five volunteers did 110 hours of work and helped thirty-six elderly people.

This agency has a very active Home Safety and Security program which is financed by the state (see chapter 4). The first $200 worth of work is always free; if the recipient has a low income the entire job is free; if the recipient has a high income he or she pays 30 percent of the remaining cost. Again, like the chore service, this program allows entry into the home so that other needs can be identified and the elderly advised of their entitlements, such as home-delivered meals.

The area agency receives donations from hospitals and individuals, and is able, at no cost to itself or to the recipients, to lend medical equipment such as hospital beds, wheelchairs, and walkers.

There is an ongoing information and referral service similar to the one described earlier. When a person is referred to another agency or service, the latter is always checked to discover whether the senior has contacted them. If this has not been done, the information and referral specialist calls the senior to find out what has happened and to offer further help. In a typical month, the service received 333 requests for information, of which 222 were first-time callers.

A sixty-five-year-old widow who lives alone was typical of the many calls I noted. She indicated that she had an income of over $5,000 a year and wanted to know what services she could receive. She was informed about Medicaid, PAAD, Life-line, and food stamps. She will be sent the necessary pamphlets and application forms, and was told that if she has any problem filling out these forms she should come into the office for assistance. If there is no contact from this woman after two weeks, a staff member will call the widow to make sure that she has received the material and understands what she must do to obtain the benefits.

A social worker contacted the area agency about a couple in their seventies with emotional problems. They had just been discharged from the hospital and needed help at home. They required assistance with food shopping, meal preparation, and housework. The information and referral specialist will send an outreach worker to their house to evaluate what services are required to enable this couple to function at home. The area agency will then make the necessary arrangements to put these services in place.

A sixty-seven-year-old widow called because her home had been broken into and she was frightened of having it happen again. She was referred to the local police department so that she could be helped under the Home Safety and Security program (see chapter 4).

The next caller was a widow in her early seventies. She lost her husband two years ago and needs to be occupied so that she will not be consumed by the loss. She feels it is very important to be out of the house each day participating in some meaningful activity. She was first referred to a volunteer job at a local nursing home but found this activity too depressing. The staff are now looking for another type of volunteer activity for her. Since the area agency feels that she also needs help coping with the loss of her husband, she is being referred to a widow support group.

An older widower called and asked if there was someone who could come to his house and spend a little time talking with him.

Arrangements are being made to have an older man from the Friendly Visitors see him for two hours once a week.

Another call was from a granddaughter who feels that her grandmother, who is seventy-seven years old and a widow, needs to get out more. This elderly lady has arthritis and is somewhat depressed. Her doctor feels that being out among people would improve both her physical and her emotional state. The area agency referred her to a nutrition site where she now gets a lunchtime hot meal, participates in group activities, and meets other older people. Since she does not drive she also gets transportation to and from the place. She attends the center twice a week and has made a few new friends. One of them now takes her shopping once a week.

An eighty-seven-year-old widow requested someone to take her shopping since she did not drive and the supermarket was not within walking distance. She was a very independent person and wanted to make her own food selections. Also, she was fairly rigid and would only shop in the middle of the week. Unfortunately, community transportation for seniors was available only on Fridays. A volunteer from the handyman-chore service was found who takes her shopping on Wednesdays.

A very simple request for help came from an eighty-four-year-old woman who is blind and whose husband is in a nursing home. She has not been able to see him in over six months since she has no one to take her there. Her only daughter lives more than fourteen hundred miles away. Since it was his birthday she particularly wanted to visit him. The area agency arranged for a volunteer to take her there and return her home after the visit. This woman is so pleased at having this service that she sent a small donation to the agency. She is now being transported once a month to the nursing home and can visit her husband regularly.

A woman in her late seventies needed some financial help in paying her transportation costs. It seems that she is a frequent user of trains and buses and is finding it too expensive. She was given information about a reduced fare program that enables her to travel at half-fare.

The last call of the morning came from a sixty-seven-year-old woman who lives alone. She needed someone to clean her house, clean the windows and kitchen cabinets, and hang her drapes. A handyman volunteer was sent to assist her with these chores. The information and referral specialist told me that the handyman program is building a fund to purchase materials to cover the cost of the repairs for those elderly who cannot afford it. The program receives many donations from those older people who have received these services.

The director of this area agency's information and referral service feels that their most important service is helping older people navigate through the system by connecting them with services that they did not know about, putting them in touch with the proper contacts, and assisting them in filling out the proper forms. In addition, she feels that the agency acts as an advocate for all the elderly in the county.

The National Association of Area Agencies on Aging has published a directory of state and area agencies on aging and a national guide for elder care information and referral (see appendices).

Other I & R Services

Although the state and area agencies on aging are the focal point of information for services and programs for the elderly, other sources are also available. Churches, other religious and ethnic organizations, family service agencies, mental health agencies, and private geriatric care managers are some possibilities. Senior centers, nutrition sites, health clinics, and hospitals are also clearinghouses for information on all kinds of programs for the elderly. National organizations like the American Association of Retired Persons (AARP) and the American Health Care Association also can be helpful (see appendices for more specific information). In addition, there are consortiums of agencies that offer information.

An example of one combined group is Info Line, an information and referral system operating in Connecticut. It is a public/private partnership that receives funds from several state departments, area agencies on aging, and the United Way. A free service operating twenty-four hours a day, it receives over eleven thousand calls a month from people seeking information or help with specific problems.[1]

Mental Health Agencies

A mental health agency in the Northeast has a specific unit that works with people sixty years of age and older. They offer a complete range of services including outreach and information and referral.

A couple in their seventies live in a lovely home with a large and attractive garden. Nine years ago, the husband had a stroke that left him with impaired mobility and speech. His wife was able to cope with his limitations and took him shopping, to social events, to the senior center, and to dine out at restaurants. Her husband was able to help with the household and garden chores.

Unfortunately, six months ago he had another stroke and now his ability to ambulate and speak is severely limited. Their only son lives too far away to be of any help. Since the husband is a well-educated man who had worked as an engineer, his impairments have severely limited his life-style and caused him to become extremely depressed. His wife came to the mental health agency for help. They arranged for him to attend a medical day-care center three times a week for six hours a day. He is transported in a chair van. Although this couple has an adequate income, their savings have been largely depleted due to their high medical expenses. The center's fees are on a sliding scale so they can afford the service.

The day-care center gives the husband the opportunity to socialize with other people, make new friends, and receive physical and speech therapy on a regular basis. In addition, the center provides help for his wife since she attends their support group for spousal caregivers. The adult day-care programs have made a marked improvement in the emotional states of both the husband and the wife and have enabled the husband, in spite of his severe handicaps, to remain at home. In addition to day care the agency arranged for a homemaker who helps the husband with bathing and transferring.

Another couple whom this agency has helped had a very different problem. They are in their early sixties and the husband is still employed as a school maintenance man. They have two sons: one lives about two hours away and the other, thirty-four years of age and retarded, lives at home with them. The mother is a housewife but had worked as a bookkeeper and seems to be far more intelligent than her husband. She began to act paranoid, accusing her husband of stealing from her, had abusive outbursts, stopped cooking and caring for the house, and generally caused disturbances in the community.

Her actions came to the attention of the police who contacted the mental health agency to help this woman. The agency made several home visits and ascertained that the wife was too ill to manage at home. They brought her to the mental health center where she was observed for two days. She was then placed in a state mental hospital where she was given a complete physical examination that revealed that there was no organic cause for her emotional problems but that she was suffering from malnutrition. She was given drug and individual therapy for six weeks. At the same time, her husband and son were also involved in therapy sessions.

The therapy plus proper nutrition improved the wife's emotional state so that her paranoia disappeared and she was able to return home after six weeks. She had to continue taking her medication. With these drugs and the support of her family, she began functioning more normally and returned to her duties as a housewife. Her other son now visits his parents more frequently and his visits also contribute to their well-being. The wife has been at home for six months now and is doing very well. She initially saw her therapist as an out-patient every week but this has been reduced to twice a month.

-※-

A sixty-nine-year-old woman had been widowed for fifteen years. She was an extremely attractive and competent person who had been working as an office manager for three prominent physicians. She led a very active life until a year ago when she had a stroke. As a result of this illness she lost the sight of one eye, and some of the function in her right arm and right leg. She could no longer drive and was forced to give up her job. The double trauma of physical disability and forced retirement produced personality changes. She became more dependent and depressed.

Although she has two married sons, with one family living in the area, this was not sufficient to make her feel better. Therefore, she herself contacted the mental health agency for help. She is now receiving psychotherapy, sees the psychiatrist every other week, and has a group therapy session twice a month. Her emotional state is much improved. She is now going out with friends, although she is still upset at not being able to drive. She is beginning to accept using public transportation and is now able to engage in some of her former activities. The mental health agency has obtained a cleaning and gardening service to help her maintain her home. In addition, they have gotten her involved with her local church which has supplied her with volunteers to help her with her food shopping. Now that she has made some progress, the agency is hoping to get her involved in some meaningful volunteer work to make up for the loss of her job.

Family Service Agencies

Family service agencies are another excellent source of information and referral and also offer many important services for the elderly. The fees are usually based on a sliding scale.

Maureen McQuire, an eighty-nine-year-old divorcée, had had four children. Unfortunately, her oldest daughter died of cancer three years ago. Maureen's children live in the same state and the youngest, a daughter, lives only four miles away and is the primary caregiver. Maureen feels that she is blessed with many grandchildren and a very supportive family. She was primarily a housewife but worked hard as a volunteer for her church. She moved into her present small house shortly after her divorce in 1956.

She had been a heavy smoker and has developed emphysema which causes her to be short of breath. In addition, she is arthritic and has difficulty getting in and out of a chair. She needs the aid of a cane for walking. In spite of these limitations she is lively and outgoing and enjoys cards, particularly bridge and gin rummy.

Her fifty-three-year-old daughter, Maureen's primary caregiver, contacted the family service agency to obtain services for her mother so that the daughter and her husband could take a vacation. This daughter helps her mother with cooking, does the laundry and the food shopping, and takes hereto the doctor. Through a local hospital's respite and renewal for caregivers program the social worker was able to supply Maureen with the care she needed while her daughter was away. In addition, she was able to relieve some of the daughter's general burden by obtaining Meals-on-Wheels, a Friendly Visitor, and a municipal service that provides transportation to medical appointments for a small fee. The agency informed the daughter that her mother was eligible for Life-Line, PAAD, and legal services, which helped relieve some of the financial burden on the family.

-※-

Jean Lewis has been a widow for twenty years. She moved into her present small house on a creek shortly before her husband died. She is eighty-five years of age and has not worked outside the home. Since her husband was a traveling salesman and they had no children, she accompanied him on his trips. She had been able to manage on her own, despite coronary-pulmonary disease, diabetes, and poor vision. However, three years ago she developed uterine cancer and has since been hospitalized several times. The visiting nurse found the house in poor condition because Jean has not been able to maintain it properly. The outside needed new siding, there were holes in the walls, the floors and kitchen linoleum needed to be replaced, and the furniture was in poor condition.

The visiting nurse who saw Jean daily to give her insulin shots and take her blood pressure contacted the family service agency for help with the repairs the house required. The nurse and the social worker made several home visits and decided that it was very important to Jean to be able to remain in her own home. Her home represented all the good things in her past life. Souvenirs, bric-a-brac, and stuffed animals that she and her husband had collected on his sales trips meant so much to her on an emotional level that her ability to continue her present living arrangement would probably lengthen her life and preserve its quality.

Although she had supportive neighbors and friends and a devoted nephew who visited her once a week, the social worker felt that in addition to the house repairs, Jean required a package of services and supervised care management. Initially, the house was repaired through a county emergency home repair program and a weatherization program. The social worker then obtained help from the county chore services to maintain Jean's home on a regular basis. A homemaker was hired to work three hours a day, twice a week. Her neighbors continued to do her shopping and the homemaker did the laundry and cleaned the house. A Friendly Visitor came to the house once a week and stayed for two hours. Jean was provided with transportation for her hospital and doctors' appointments.

In general, the family service worker arranged for a network of services for this very disabled woman. She herself visited Jean at least twice a month to see how well she was functioning. If not for this ongoing supervision, Jean would have had to be placed in a nursing home and would not have lived as long or remained in as good shape as she did. With medical treatment and agency support she was able to keep her semi-independent life-style for three more years. She died recently at the age of 88 in her own home.

Geriatric Care Managers

The type of service that Jean Lewis received is called geriatric care management, a relatively new concept that has become more available in the past five or six years. This kind of care is offered by some private nonprofit agencies such as family service agencies, but is more usually supplied by private for-profit groups. In addition to information and referral, these agencies offer a complete array of social, psychological, and health-care services to families. Geriatric care managers are used mainly by adult children with aging parents, particularly those who live at a distance. The agencies serve as substitute caregivers for the younger relatives. They assess the older parents' needs and tailor programs to enable these elderly people to live independently in their own homes.

> The private geriatric care manager is a professional with a graduate degree in the field of human services (Social Work, Psychology, Gerontology) or a substantial equivalent (i.e., RN) certified or licensed at the independent practice level of his or her state or profession, who is duly trained and experienced in the assessment, coordination, monitoring and direct delivery of services to the elderly and their families.[2]

In 1986, the National Association of Private Geriatric Care Managers was formed and there are now 225 member agencies throughout the country.

A middle-aged couple recently moved in with the husband's mother who is eighty-six years old and lives alone in a five-bedroom house. She has edema in both legs, arthritis, and the beginning of senile dementia. She has difficulty walking and becomes easily confused. The son did not want to place his mother in a nursing home nor did she want to leave her home of many years. Therefore, he and his wife were willing to live with her and offer her support and care. However, the wife had a long commute and did not get home until late in the evening, and the son's job required him to travel extensively.

Because he was at home so infrequently and not really able to care for her, the son contacted a private geriatric care manager to oversee a program of services for his mother. This professional arranged for a home health aide to come to the house each morning from 7:00 to 9:00 A.M. and help her get dressed and give her breakfast. She was enrolled in an adult day-care center that she attended five days a week. The day-care center transported her in a van that picked her up when the aide left and returned her home at the end of the day. The son and daughter-in-law were also referred to a respite program that gave them relief from caring for the mother and allowed them to get away for an occasional weekend or short vacation.

-✳-

Tricia, a woman in her mid-thirties, asked her boss for the following day off. She told him, "My grandmother's being released from the hospital. She's just over pneumonia, and she's still pretty weak. I'd like to get her settled down at home and meet the home health aides who are going to take care of her."

Her boss knew that Tricia had driven the two-hundred-mile round trip several evenings recently to see her eighty-six-year-old grandmother. She also knew that Tricia's mother had Alzheimer's disease and was being cared for by her husband in their retirement home in Arizona and that the grandmother depended on Tricia as the closest relative. Separated from her husband and with a six-year-old son, Tricia seemed near the breaking point. Therefore, her boss readily agreed to her request for time off.

After Tricia returned to work she wept and said, "Poor dear. It's taken a terrible toll on her. Her memory's been affected, and she's very frail and weak. I don't think she'll ever be the same again, and she knows it. The worst part is, she's terrified of being sent to a nursing home."

Fortunately, Tricia explained, her grandmother had enough money to pay for care at home and had given Tricia power of attorney. "What I've done is to hand the whole business over to a new agency here. The people who run it call themselves 'geriatric care managers.' They'll do anything from hiring a housekeeper to packing and moving an older person to a new place. A friend of mine who is a graduate social worker started the agency with two friends who were hospital geriatric care workers."

Tricia said they had arranged for a health-care service near her grandmother's home to supply round-the-clock aides for two weeks. The agency would maintain contact and evaluate the invalid's progress during that time. Meanwhile, they had listed her grandmother's fine old brick house, which is in a respectable neighborhood, with a home-share matching agency in the area.

"Even when Granny's well enough to manage without the health aides, she's going to need someone there at night—if not for her sake then for mine," Tricia added. "I'm not sure how she'll feel about sharing her home. But it's certainly large enough. And I think I can persuade her that she needs a companion if she wants to continue living there."

The geriatric care managers would screen the home-share candidates' applications and set up interviews for Tricia with those deemed suitable. She planned to introduce the person she approved of to her grandmother. Tricia also counted on the agency to engage housekeeping help and to serve as a liaison with the home-sharing agency, which would be monitoring the arrangement.

"If it works out the way I hope it will, it'll be a tremendous relief for me. I'll call Granny often, of course, and drive up with my little boy for a weekend once a month or so. And in the meantime I can try to get on with my life," Tricia finished with a sigh.[3]

In this chapter and chapter 6 I have been discussing the many agencies and organizations, public and private, profit and nonprofit, that offer a variety of services to assist the elderly to remain in their own homes. I have also given some examples of programs that can help maintain or improve the quality of life for them.

Older people can relocate to other parts of the country and find a new house or apartment to continue with their independent lifestyle. There are many reasons for doing this, all of which will be explored in the next chapter.

The Sun Shines Bright

Relocating to a Warmer Climate

The most common reasons for relocating are to live in a warm climate and to be near children or other close family members. In the former case, older people tend to move from the Northeast and the Midwest to Florida, Arizona, California, Texas, and North Carolina. Florida has attracted the largest number of elderly in-migrants from Connecticut, Indiana, New Jersey, New York, Ohio, and Pennsylvania.[1] The elderly who can afford two homes are called "snowbirds." They continue to maintain their homes in the North and spend the winter months in the South. Many of them are planning to eventually relocate permanently to their winter homes.

Sylvia and Tom, a couple in their mid-seventies, have been married for fifty-two years. Thirty-four years ago they bought a house in a suburban area in the Northeast. When this home became difficult to maintain a few years ago they moved to a small apartment in a nearby city.

They began finding the cold winters unpleasant and started spending part of this season in Florida. After doing this for three years, which involved "scurrying around for a new rental each year," they decided to look for a small house of their own. For the past three years they have been coming to Florida for five months and living in a condominium unit in an adult community.

Although when they bought this condominium apartment they considered themselves to be snowbirds, they now feel it would make a good permanent residence in a few years. Interestingly, although it was Tom who hates the cold and who initiated spending the winters in a warm climate, it is Sylvia who is now more ready to give up the apartment in the North and become a regular southern resident.

The condominium unit consists of a kitchen, living-dining room with an L-shaped den, screened porch (which they enclosed in glass), one bedroom, and two baths. They both selected this home because "it was unpretentious, in a semirural setting, and was relatively inexpensive."

In addition, for Sylvia, "this community looked like 'home' and reminded me of my childhood and the place where I grew up. I like the feeling of country and the fact that each apartment overlooks a grassy area and a canal. I love looking at water. The community offers many amenities: a clubhouse, swimming pool, library, exercise rooms, evening entertainments, and classes in nutrition, dancing, painting, and health education. There is also free bus transportation three times a week to supermarkets and shopping malls."

Sylvia tends to be more involved in the retirement community while Tom is more of a private person and a loner. He spends much time in the home doing repairs, and painting and refinishing secondhand furniture they have bought. He also tends a small garden in the front and back of their apartment. He is an avid reader, particularly of spy stories and mysteries. They both like to watch old movies on their VCR and rent video cassettes from the library.

Sylvia, on the other hand, is very involved in their housing community and in the larger community. She attends a watercolor class, health club, and exercise program. She has joined the residence volunteers and works at least twice a month for the library, hospice, and cancer groups. Because of her education and professional experience, Sylvia was readily accepted as a volunteer at a home for troubled teenagers. She volunteers her time one day a week and provides individual counseling and supervision of some of the regular staff.

Each morning, at 7:00 or 7:30, they take a brisk walk around the community and enjoy greeting the other residents who are also engaged in this activity. They like this feeling of comraderie; Sylvia calls it a "walkership." In the evenings they attend concerts, theater, and movies, which are very accessible. Also, there is a medical center immediately adjacent to their housing complex. They are most pleased with this convenient health service and have found a doctor and a dentist that they both like.

They both attended an institute for retired people and took a course in musical comedy last year. They entertain guests from the North occasionally and take them to the local museums and on sightseeing trips in the area.

One of the things that has particularly pleased both of them is the casual but solid relationships they share with their neighbors. When someone goes food shopping, he or she will invariably check with neighbors to see if they need anything from the store. If Tom and Sylvia want company for dining out, they can usually find someone to go with them. Recently, before Sylvia and Tom left on a trip, one of their neighbors asked them to dinner since she felt they might not have enough food left or be too tired to cook. Their only negative comment concerned the community's constant card playing which did not interest them. In addition, Tom is somewhat annoyed by pressure from the other residents to become more involved in the community.

There is an additional reason for this couple's move to Florida: Sylvia's older sister and her husband live permanently in this state, although about 150 miles away. They have been spending Thanksgiving and the Christmas holidays together and Sylvia and Tom spend a few days with her sister and brother-in-law on the way down and on the way back from the South. Since Sylvia and Tom have no children and Tom has no siblings, this sister and brother-in-law are their closest relatives.

Sylvia and Tom's small one-bedroom apartment in a northern city is centrally located, and they can walk to the library and convenience stores. There is free bus transportation every day: three round trips during the day and one in the evening. In the building itself, there is an ice cream store, a restaurant, a video store, and a dry cleaners. Although they like their two homes, Sylvia is the more enthusiastic about their life in the North. She feels stimulated and says, "I feel younger and more vigorous in the North than I do in Florida and I like living in an intergenerational apartment building. I feel more alive in the city. I don't have the same excitement about living in Florida." But she added, "I find Florida very pleasant and I feel extremely peaceful here."

Now that they have spent five months each year for the past three years in their home in Florida, they feel they made a good decision. Tom likes getting away from the cold and is enjoying the relaxation, warmth, and easy-going life-style in the South. But since he is now living in an age-segregated community, he is irritated by the more elderly residents who are often slow and cautious in their walking and driving. He said, "I can't stand their creepiness." However, Sylvia does not think that being surrounded by other older people is a "downer." In fact, she said, "I feel proud of them and enjoy seeing beautiful older people who are active and busy."

Although they can afford to maintain their two homes, they are beginning to find the shuttling back and forth each year getting to be a chore and anticipate that they will no longer be able to do this without a great deal of difficulty in a few years. This reason for relocating to Florida on a permanent basis was repeated by many of the other snowbirds.

-✸-

Now we will meet a number of couples who have found a permanent residence in the South.

Judith and Manny are in their mid-sixties and have been married for forty-six years. They have three sons and six grandchildren who live in the Northeast. When Judith and Manny lived in the North their children and their families lived close by.

Manny was an accountant who acted as a consultant to a number of nonprofit organizations such as small art museums. Judith was only a high school graduate when she married but decided to return to school while she was raising her family. She obtained B.A. and M.A. degrees and obtained a job as a guidance counselor when her youngest child was ten.

Judith and Manny met when they were quite young and married in their early twenties. They were fairly radical in their youth and worked hard for left-wing causes. Judith helped her PTA desegregate the school in the early 1950s, and both are still active in fighting for civil rights.

When the children were young, they had only a modest income, and would take inexpensive vacations with them, such as camping and nature hikes. They had a very large circle of friends, whom they saw frequently. They spent much of their leisure time listening to music and reading. Manny's major hobby is photography and he has his own darkroom. Their home is decorated with many of his framed photographs. They both are fanatical exercisers. They used to jog and swim, but they have given up the former and are now avid walkers. Manny walks twenty miles a week, and Judith uses her exercise bicycle every day. They also are members of a health club, and do indoor swimming.

Their last residence in the North was a two-story, three-bedroom, two-bath townhouse. Manny retired two years ago and Judith retired a year later. Shortly after, they sold their townhouse, packed their bags, and moved into a short-term rental in Florida. Within a month, they were able to buy a house. They now reside in a three-bedroom, two-bath condominium in an adult community.

Manny cited the financial advantage of living in Florida as the main reason for the move. He said, "We could manage in the North but we could live a hellavu lot better in Florida. We sold our home for almost three times what we paid for our present condominium. Our taxes were eight times higher than what they are here. And since inflation is going to make that difference even larger in the future, the economics of living in Florida will be more attractive. So now we don't have to watch our expenses so carefully and can live much easier here."

They both agreed that their second reason for relocating was that they like to exercise and the Florida weather allows them to do outdoor activities all year round.

They felt that their ability to find a new home and adjust so quickly and so well was "due to the fact that we've moved so many times—we've made at least eight moves and this will be our ninth." Judith added, "We have learned to settle in quickly since we have made so many moves. Also, we're not savers." In addition to their regular residence they owned a vacation house in the mountains for twelve years. They sold it six years ago because maintaining two homes was becoming too much of a burden.

Their other reasons for moving to Florida were that they had many friends who were snowbirds who had settled in the area, and they did not want to be too far away from their children and other close family. This ruled out the West coast and the Southwest. In addition, one of their sons has a mother-in-law who lives nearby so he and his wife can now see both sets of parents on the same trip. Since their move, Manny and Judith have been back North for a week at Thanksgiving, and a week in January. They plan to return in the summer when they will stay one week at a son's house, a month in a rented apartment in New York City, and a week visiting friends in Massachusetts.

They enjoy entertaining friends and family from the North. In addition to the snowbirds they already knew, they have made many new friends. People had given them the names of friends and relatives to contact and many of their meetings have worked out very well for them. They are friendly with their neighbors but cautious about becoming too close since they have such a wide circle of friends outside the adult community. Also they feel that "if you get too friendly with your neighbors and you have a falling out, it can become too unpleasant since you can't avoid seeing them."

Their present life-style is a continuation of their former outdoor activities. They walk five to six days a week, and cover three miles in forty-three minutes. Judith swims laps in the pool every day. They have joined the adult community's tennis club, but so far have not found the time to play. They have attended the local university's music classes and Judith is now taking a course in "the new world" once a week. Manny is writing a family history for his grandchildren and works with a large computer set up in his study.

They are both active volunteers, mainly outside their adult community. However, Judith is participating in "We Care," which provides the residents with transportation for medical appointments. Manny is active in the county council on the arts, where he helps small companies with their budgets, long-range plans, advertising, and marketing. He works as a volunteer consultant at least once a week. His town is reconstructing an old school building into a town cultural center and he will be arranging their art exhibitions.

They are both active volunteers at a national wildlife refuge center and work eight hours a month at the visitor's center. By next year, they hope to be knowledgeable enough to take groups on tours through the site. They are now reading, walking, and attending lectures to learn more about the refuge center.

Judith has joined the local chapter of NOW and attends meetings when she can. She plans to move slowly but anticipates taking a more active role in the near future. She said, "We do miss the theater and will be exploring a series of plays that are being produced locally by a repertory company."

They are both fortunate that they are in good health. Manny did have knee surgery due to his injuries in his youth. However, this does not seem to interfere with any of his activities.

They both confessed that "if we were rich enough to afford an apartment in midtown Manhattan and attendance at a health club, we would have chosen to move to the city rather than to relocate to Florida." However, they like living in a year-round summer climate and said, "The heat doesn't bother us. In the warmer months we walk early in the mornings. We don't find the beach too hot, and can run in and out of the ocean to cool off. Also, our house, our car, and all the places are air-conditioned."

Judith misses her children and grandchildren and also the old friends they left behind. However, with their trips to the North and their sons' visits to the South, they spend about as much time with them as before their move. Interestingly, their youngest son found his parents' move as difficult as it had been initially for them.

Now that they are living in their new home they are convinced that they made the correct decision in moving to Florida. However, they each have a slight problem adjusting to seeing so many elderly on the streets, in the library, and in the stores. They miss not seeing other age groups. Manny said, "I would prefer a less age-segregated environment. That's one reason why we chose to do volunteering so that we could see and work with some younger people. Also I would prefer to live in a mixed ethnic and racial community."

Judith summed up her feelings about Florida by saying, "It is so cheerful and pleasant to have so many warm sunny days. And this is even more significant after you are retired."

-✳-

Another couple, Nancy and Jim, were at odds with each other about moving away from their home in the North. He wanted very much to live in a warm climate and was not upset at leaving children behind while she preferred to remain in her house. In addition, she said, "I could not move while our fifteen-year-old dog and my mother-in-law were still alive. Neither would have survived the move."

About five years ago, close friends of Nancy and Jim relocated to Florida and invited them to visit their new house. Nancy was favorably impressed with their living arrangements and decided that she would explore houses in the area. Four years ago, after both her mother-in-law and the dog had died, Nancy suggested that they take a trial run in Florida and rent a house for three months and see how they liked it.

Jim really enjoyed life in Florida, and soon began to pressure his wife about buying a house. They found one they liked in a new adult community. It has two bedrooms, two baths, a living room that opens into a dining room, a kitchen, and an enclosed porch. The community is attractively landscaped and their apartment overlooks the golf course. It is well located, with the pool and clubhouse only a short block away.

Nancy and Jim had lived in their former house their entire married life. Three of their sons live in the same area and the fourth lives in the Midwest. One has never been married; the other three have been divorced and two have remarried. Nancy and Jim have six grandchildren.

Jim is a high school graduate and worked as an outside salesman. About thirty years ago, he had a silent heart attack and subsequently became overly concerned about his health and began to have anxiety attacks. He participated in group therapy and eventually became less apprehensive. However, he was only able to make a marginal living so Nancy was forced to return to work. A college graduate, she obtained a job as a high school teacher from which she finally retired six years ago. Jim lost his sales lines and finally took work as a salesperson in a hardware store. Since their joint income was insufficient to support a family of six, Nancy had to take a second job at night as an instructor at a local college.

Nancy is an extremely attractive and energetic woman. Even when she worked she was active in the PTA, Boy Scouts, and the sisterhood at her temple. After her retirement, she took courses in sculpture and bridge, and now plays bridge socially two or three times a week.

Jim developed emphysema and some heart problems and was forced to retire on disability. Since his wife had two jobs he stayed home and took care of the household chores in addition to the repairs and the outside work. His main interest was gardening. He functioned well as a house husband until he was involved in a terrible accident about ten years ago.

A friend who was visiting and had parked his station wagon in their driveway had a propane gas tank in the back of the wagon. Apparently it leaked and the car filled with gas. Jim was helping his friend carry out some packages to the car. When the friend put his key in the lock to open the door, the static electricity caused the gas trapped in the car to ignite. The wagon exploded with pieces flying all over the area. Jim was thrown across the lawn, with bits of glass on his face. The noise of the explosion punctured his eardrums and now he has to wear a hearing aid. Moreover, the trauma aggravated his negative emotional state and he began to suffer serious depression.

This weakened condition made it difficult for Jim to continue to take care of the repairs and the gardening. He found this extremely frustrating and became very upset at not being able to do the two things he liked best. It became apparent that they would have to sell their home and move to a condominium. But Nancy discovered that making this desirable move was not so simple: "When we looked at the condos in the area we found that we could not afford them. They were selling for much more than what we could get for our house."

Since the care of the house became too difficult for Jim and they could not afford to buy a condo in the North, Jim began to push for a move to the South. "I was finding the cold winters very difficult and really wanted to live in a warmer climate," he said. Three years ago they found a condo selling at a reasonable price and two and a half years ago moved into their Florida home.

"We got rid of all our furniture with the exception of two night tables, two lamps, a TV set, a bed, and an étagère. I wanted to make a new beginning since we had picked our unit from a floor plan and it would be brand-new. I was surprised at how easy the move was although I did feel a little funny about leaving the kids," Nancy explained. She went on to say, "Although I would have preferred to continue to live in the North, once we had bought the new condo I found myself looking forward to the move. I became very involved with furnishing and decorating our new home."

Jim added, "I feel that we were very lucky to have picked this community since everyone is so friendly and warm here." They both felt that they have been leading a most relaxed life here in contrast to the more hectic existence in the North.

Nancy said, "And we have made so many new friends, at least thirty, whom we entertain after dinner with coffee and cake, play cards, or eat out at a restaurant. I really enjoy not getting up to the tune of an alarm clock, not that I really sleep late since I want to enjoy all this marvelous sunshine. I swim forty-six laps in the pool every morning and get Jim to walk back and forth around the pool while I'm doing my laps."

Although they socialize as a couple, Nancy is the more active of the two and is involved in many separate activities. She does water aerobics, takes an exercise class, does tap dancing and line dancing, and plays bridge. She also meditates for twenty minutes in the morning and in the evening. Jim plays poker and they both participate in the once-a-month chartered bus trips to the theater. When they first moved in they served as cochairmen of the program committee for one year. Now Jim is president of their section of the condominium association.

"We're busy all the time but it's hard to say what we do. I enjoy the fact the sun is shining all the time. The sun is my tranquilizer. Both of us enjoy Florida. Even when it rains it doesn't last too long. We visit our children in the North twice a year, and my family in the Midwest at least that often. One of our sons has an office in Florida and so he stops in to see us every few months. Another one of our sons visits us each Easter. We do most of this traveling in the three summer months since we find it a little too hot at that time in Florida," Nancy offered.

She confessed that although she does miss the change of seasons, she likes the sun and the nice weather and the fact that you can be outdoors all the time. Although, as she had told me earlier, she had not found making this move too difficult, it took her a whole year before she referred to Florida as her home.

Jim had only positive things to say about their move to Florida. "I feel that this is the ideal situation for us. Since I could no longer take care of a house we needed to live in a condo arrangement. It is so much less expensive to buy and maintain a condo unit here. Also moving into a new community makes it so much easier to make friends, since everyone is in the same boat. There is more than enough to keep us busy and happy. This life-style is not only pleasurable but adds years to your life. I like the sociability and it's so easy to talk to people here." He does not share his wife's feeling of missing their grandchildren. He said, "Grandchildren are wonderful to visit but not for too long at a time. After a week of being with them, I go out of my mind." Jim feels that they actually spend more quality time with their children since they tend to see them separately rather than in a large group at family functions and holidays.

Jim ended the interview by saying, "It took me two years to convince my wife to move to Florida. I don't miss the North one bit particularly since so many of our friends had moved away. This was the best decision I've made!"

-⚜-

Renee and Frank are a very interesting couple who not only chose living in the South because of the climate but actually enjoy the heat in the summer. Frank is sixty-five and Renee is ten years younger; their marriage is the second for both. They have been married for ten years and appear to be extremely happy together. Their first marriages were extremely poor and ended in divorce for both of them.

Frank has three children and five grandchildren and Renee has two children. They all live in the Northeast with the exception of one of Renee's sons who lives in the Northwest. Renee and Frank met at a meeting of Parents without Partners and liked each other immediately.

They both described themselves as very different when they were younger but each through his or her own efforts changed into happier and better functioning people. Renee explained, "I was a shrinking violet, I never had much self-respect. The best thing that happened to me was when my first husband became an alcoholic and I was forced to reevaluate my life. I joined Alanon, a group for people with a family member who is an alcoholic. This group was extremely helpful and I became a much better person. I developed self-esteem and realized that I was worth something."

Renee went on to say that her new self-image allowed her to attend a meeting of the League of Women Voters at her neighbor's suggestion, something she would not have been able to do previously. She really enjoyed discussing local and state government and current events. She said, "I was fascinated. It turned me on like crazy. I couldn't get enough of it. The first year I was very quiet and merely listened. But after that I joined one of the committees and developed enough self-confidence to lead a workshop." In addition to this activity, she joined a class in international folk dancing, an interest she has continued to pursue for the past twenty years.

Frank described himself as an introvert who decided to make himself into a more outgoing person. He said, "I read many books on this subject and made a plan with specific time frames for achieving certain goals. I joined organizations and forced myself to get up on the floor and ask a question. Next I would try to enter into the discussion. Once finding myself comfortable in these roles I went a step further and joined a committee and eventually served as chairman."

Although he claims that he was very nervous at first, he became so adept that he ran for office successfully as district leader. He later made a run for state senator but was defeated. However, he thoroughly enjoyed this experience and is now fairly skilled at making speeches and meeting new people.

This couple enjoy outdoor activities and are excellent swimmers. Fifteen years ago, Frank learned how to scuba dive and has become an enthusiast. He introduced Renee to this sport, and she now thoroughly enjoys it. In fact, they are planning to celebrate their tenth wedding anniversary by taking a trip to the Caribbean for scuba diving.

They each had moved into apartments after their respective divorces. When they married, they shared a new apartment and then bought a small ranch house. Frank had a B.A. degree; twenty-five years later he obtained a M.A. in education. He did this because he was extremely interested in the subject but did not intend to use this degree to pursue a vocation. He worked in the family business and when it was sold he continued to work for the new owners for another two years. He retired five years ago.

Shortly after Frank's retirement they began to think of relocating to the South. Renee had always liked Florida; she had made frequent visits to this state because her mother lives there. In fact her mother is still alive at 101. Renee now is able to see her mother almost every other afternoon.

They were very systematic in looking for a house and knew that they wanted a separate unit on one level that was airy and light, offered complete privacy, and had an attached garage. They were also looking for a location in an adult community that had a large swimming pool and an active clubhouse with evening programs. They found a lovely house that fulfilled all of their requirements. It has a large eat-in kitchen, with an open wall to the dining-living room, a master bedroom and bath at one end, and a smaller bedroom and bath at the other end of the house. In addition, they added three sliding glass doors to the large screened porch, making it useable in the summer heat.

They are very happy living in Florida all year. Their reasons for selecting this state as their new home have proved correct. Aside from Renee's desire to be near her elderly mother, they both knew that they not only could stand the hot summer weather but also really liked it.

Frank said, "Our house in the North had escalated in price so that with the additional money we were able to purchase a really nice home in Florida. The cost of housing, maintenance, and taxes were much lower in this state. In addition I disliked the cold intensively. Because of our interest in swimming and scuba diving we wanted to live near a large body of water. Also, in south Florida you can swim all year round." Frank's only concession to getting older is that he now restricts his diving to water less than fifty feet deep.

Renee and Frank lead a very active life. He plays tennis and swims almost daily. He is vice president of the tennis club and plays doubles in the local tournaments. He is involved in the civic association and has been both education chairman and program chairman, and is now the president. In addition, he has worked on the last presidential campaign and is a county committeeman.

She also swims laps in the pool daily and spends three hours, three times a week, at the gym. She starts at 6:45 in the morning. She plays duplicate bridge twice a week, and takes courses in ballroom dancing, current events, and ceramics once a week. She is a member of the community's beautification committee.

In addition to their separate activities, they do many things together. They have subscriptions to the ballet, music and dance programs at the local university, and a repertory theater group.

Before they moved south they did not know anybody who lived there with the exception of Frank's brother who had moved to the same town two years before. Now they have found many new friends in their adult community and some of their northern friends have started to spend the winters in Florida. They return to the North at Thanksgiving and in July each year to see their children and grandchildren. Their children visit them about once a year. Renee says, "I love to have them here in Florida and I also enjoy having lots of other overnight guests."

On balance, Frank is completely satisfied with his move to Florida. On the other hand, Renee says, "I guess I'm 85 percent satisfied. I love the outdoors, the swimming and scuba diving, and this marvelous warm climate. But I love to cook and bake and find the food shopping not adequate so that I have to import special products from the North."

More important, Renee misses her children and one very close friend. She said, "This was the hardest—leaving my children and this friend behind. Also, I feel that our grandchildren are missing a lot by not being able to see us more than once or twice a year." Except for these reservations, she does feel it was a good move and expects to be able to continue to live in this house for at least the next twenty years.

-✵-

A charming and erudite couple, Terry and Fred, were married fifteen years ago. This was a second marriage for both. He had been widowed and she had been divorced for the second time shortly before they met. Fred related the story of how they met. "I was very depressed after my first wife died. She had been very ill with cancer for two years and we had to move back to the city so that she could be close to the hospital where she was treated on an out-patient basis. After she died, my friends were concerned about my emotional state and were busily introducing me to their single women friends. I was not really interested and continued to feel lonely. Terry had a concert series with a couple we both knew and couldn't use her ticket one Saturday night. She told them to give it to someone since she had to be out of town that weekend. I enjoyed the concert very much and when my friends described Terry I thought I would like to meet her."

At this point, Terry interjected, "Darling, let me finish the story. He called me the next morning to tell me how much he had enjoyed using my ticket. And invited me for lunch so that he could properly thank me. I accepted and we spent a very pleasant day together. The next morning I received another phone call from him and this time he proposed marriage. I was a bit nonplused, to put it mildly, and suggested that we should get to know each other first. Fred was a most attentive and persistent suitor and we did get married some months later—a decision I have never regretted."

Fred is in his mid-eighties and Terry in her early seventies. He had been a distinguished college professor, writer, performer, and composer, and she had worked in a city school system as a teacher, vocational counselor, and assistant principal. After she retired, she studied psychotherapy and became a certified therapist before they moved to Florida in 1977. Terry's mother was still alive at that time and she moved with them. They placed her in a residential hotel; since she was quite frail Terry had to be her primary caregiver. During this time Terry was too busy with her mother to be involved in any outside activities. Her mother died a year and a half later.

Terry and Fred moved to Florida twelve years ago. At first they rented an apartment but when the rent increased dramatically they decided to buy a condominium in an apartment building. They have been living for the past twelve years in a very large, attractive three-bedroom, two-and-a-half bath unit with a huge balcony that overlooks a beautiful garden and fountain. They enjoy their Florida home very much. Terry said, "Shortly after we moved in we were invited to an in-house cocktail party to meet the other residents. Everyone is most friendly here and we have excellent neighbors. In fact we became so close to two of them that they became like family. They have just recently passed away and I miss them dreadfully."

Before Terry and Fred met they each had been exploring moving from the Northeast to a warmer climate. Terry is very prone to upper respiratory infections and has had the flu and pneumonia several times in the cold weather. Her doctor had recommended that she live in the South. She had looked into California and Florida. She visited her brother in the latter state and liked the area. Fred and his first wife had spent vacations in California, Arizona, and Florida. Although he liked California, he thought it was too far away from the East coast and his family. He did not find Arizona attractive and said, "Florida seemed the most comfortable of the southern states. In fact, my daughter-in-law says that this is as close to paradise as you'll ever get."

They both like living here very much, although Terry was more attached than her husband to her former home in the North. However, she says, "I like living in this climate. And it's surprisingly comfortable even in the summer, since we live right on the ocean where it's ten degrees cooler than inland. Every place is air-conditioned and the ocean breezes are delightful. It's just gorgeous here in the warm weather!"

Like so many other couples who have chosen to relocate, they are very active people. Terry used to swim competitively and now swims in the ocean and does laps in the pool daily. Fred also uses the pool regularly, but he does not like the sand on the beach and does not join her in the ocean. He also takes long walks every day.

Although Fred is getting on in years and has arthritis, he has a very good sense of humor and says with a twinkle, "Every morning is a new adventure. I wake up with a new ache or pain." This does not stop him from doing his physical activities; in fact, he feels better after his exercise. In addition to his chronic condition, he has glaucoma in one eye. However, he is still able to drive a car during daylight hours. Fred had been a professional violinist and had played in a symphony orchestra. He continued to practice on this instrument until six years ago when his arthritis forced him to stop. He now plays the piano at least forty-five minutes each day to keep his fingers and hands nimble.

Fred said, "Staying intellectually alive is most important." He and his wife both live according to this maxim. They attend concerts, lectures, ballet, theater, and museums on a regular basis. Their major activity, which they do as volunteers, is working for an institute at a local college. This institute offers older people courses on an informal, noncredit basis on such subjects as psychology, biology, philosophy, literature, art, and investments. The students pay a modest fee and the instructors are all retired professionals. The classes are held three afternoons a week from late October through April.

This institute has been in existence for fifteen years, but Terry and Fred became involved several years after it had started. They both have been teaching courses in their respective disciplines. In addition, Terry served as curriculum coordinator and this is her second year as president of the board of directors. This is a very responsible job since the institute has over six thousand students.

Terry and Fred are close to their families and travel all over the country several times a year, attending graduations and weddings or just visiting their children and grandchildren. Fred said, "In addition, we used to take annual trips to different parts of the world. In the past five years, I have found this too tiring and we take shorter trips only. I have been spending summers at an institute in the western part of New York State for the past forty-six years and after we were married Terry has joined me. I hope I never have to give that up."

They have found that the Florida climate has been extremely beneficial to their respective physical conditions. Terry has been fairly free of flu and pneumonia and Fred is in much less pain from his arthritis and now walks fairly upright and without a limp. He says, "When I leave the North after a visit with one of the children, I start feeling better as soon as I board the plane. When I arrive in Florida and start peeling off the layers of my clothes, I just love it!"

-※※-

The couples we have met all moved to Florida primarily because of the warm climate. However, there is another major reason for relocating and that is to live close to family members, particularly children and grandchildren. Remember Renee's remark about how much she missed seeing her grandchildren and how much she felt they were losing by not having their grandparents close by? Our next couple's decision to move was due to the fact that their only grandchild lived so far away that they could only see her a few times a year.

During the forty-three years of their marriage, Rose and Hal had moved five times—more frequently in the early years—and each move had been an upgrade in house and property. After the first rented room and then a small apartment in New York City, they moved out to the suburbs. The three houses they had lived in were all in the New York metro area—not because of any special loyalty to their native city, but because of the increasing dependence of Hal's mother.

The year his mother died, Hal turned sixty-seven. Unsettling changes at the company where he had worked for almost twenty-three years induced him to think seriously, if reluctantly, about retirement. All this followed on the heels of grandparenthood; their daughter's child had been born the year before.

Being a grandmother was a long-awaited joy for Rose and she wanted to see the baby as often as possible, so she and Hal made the trip to North Carolina as often as they could—every six to eight weeks—using all their vacation time this way. On some of those visits, they spent time looking at houses in the area—casually at first, then more purposefully. In spite of their love for their home of twenty-two years in the Northeast, they recognized that their circumstances were changing and they would have to make some changes, too.

The realization that a move would be good for them did not

strike suddenly. It involved a balancing of pros and cons. For Rose, it meant leaving not just a lovely house, but the community with its familiar people and organizations. Although Hal's attachment to his place of employment (30 miles away) was much stronger than his attachment to the town he lived in, he, too, had grown used to the familiar conveniences (stores, medical offices, etc.). Much more important, another child, a single son living in the city, would be left behind, as would Rose's mother and three sisters.

The main argument on the pro side was the advantage of being closer to their daughter and her family. Rose and Hal felt they could be of help to the young couple and could count on them if the need arose. They also knew that it would become more and more difficult to make frequent long-distance visits and they wanted to be more than absentee grandparents.

Many other reasons persuaded Rose and Hal of the wisdom of a move south: the wish to live in a warmer climate, in a community with lower living costs, in a livelier (several universities and a large research-industrial park) but less densely populated area (New York area traffic had become intolerable), and in a smaller, easier-to-care-for house.

Rose had an additional motive; she thought it would be an excellent diversion for Hal, keeping him occupied so that he would have little time to brood over his retirement. She also reasoned that her own life had become somewhat static while all about her changes were taking place. Old friends and neighbors moved away, stores closed or moved, doctors and dentists retired, and clubs disbanded. Her house seemed to grow larger each time she vacuumed or mopped floors, and all the extra space only served as storage for accumulated junk and children's belongings that had never been claimed.

Greater distance from their son, and other family members and friends, would mean less frequent visits, but Hal and Rose expected that they could keep in touch by mail, by phone, and by occasional visits. As for their son, he had often declared his intention of moving away from the New York area, and without family responsibilities he could easily do this at any time.

After all these things had been considered, the benefits appeared to outweigh the drawbacks and Rose and Hal began to look forward to the adventure of living in another part of the country for the first time in their lives. Of course, it was not a strange place, but one that had become familiar to them over the dozen years of their daughter's residence there. Rose concluded, "What the future holds I cannot know, but this move to North Carolina seems the best choice for us at this time."

—※—

For Sandra and Bill a move to the South was also partly motivated by a desire to be close to a family member. This time it was not to be near a child, but to be close to Sandra's sister and her husband. As it turned out, very fortuitously, one of their two daughters, because of her husband's job, moved to a location about an hour away from their new home in Florida. So now they are close to both a sister and a daughter, and more recently a grandchild as well.

They have led a rather interesting life because Bill's professorship at a large metropolitan college enabled him to take research fellowships and sabbaticals that led to travel in the United States, Europe, and Asia. Prior to her marriage and before her children were born, Sandra worked in an advertising agency but remained at home after that and raised their two daughters.

They lived in a small, compact two-story house very close to the college where Bill worked. Because of his schedule, he was able to come home for lunch almost every day and spend time with the family. This was another reason why it was difficult for Sandra to work outside the home. For intellectual stimulation, she tried to go to the metropolitan area once a week where she met friends and went to museums and art galleries. She loved to read and wanted to pass this pleasure on to her children. Therefore, she spent a good deal of time at the library with them.

She has learned to knit and sew. Although she has taken courses in painting and sculpture she has not continued with these interests because she does not feel that she has any talent. She attended functions at the college and did join the faculty wives club. But she added, "I'm not a joiner or a volunteer. I find it hard to deal with groups of people I don't really know."

When the children were young, Sandra wanted to purchase a house in the country that they could use first for summer vacations and later as a retirement residence. However, Bill did not want to maintain two homes and so they rented houses in a nearby mountain area. After the children were grown, they began renting a house for three to four months in a New England college town and have been doing this for the past nine years.

Five years ago, at age seventy, Bill retired as a professor of mathematics. They decided to spend the winter in Florida and found a place to rent in Sandra's sister's adult community. Bill really liked the climate and the ability to be outdoors every day, since he was interested in walking, biking, and playing raquetball. When he was younger, he was an avid handball player, jogger, skier, rollerskater, hiker, biker, and camper. Sandra was not interested in athletics and spent much of her time indoors reading. However, she liked spending time with her sister daily.

Bill became insistent that they buy a condominium unit in Florida and make it their permanent residence. Sandra agreed with the decision to buy a winter house in Florida but she said, "I hate the extremely hot and humid summers and wanted to own another home in a cool area in the Northeast and make it our main home." However, Bill's wishes prevailed and four years ago they sold their house and moved to Florida. They bought a small two-bedroom condo in her sister's development and continue to rent a house in New England from the end of May through the beginning of October. Next summer they are thinking of spending the time in the Northwest where their other daughter and her husband live.

Sandra told me, "I like missing the New York winters and I enjoy being in Florida during those four or five months. It has been extremely helpful to my sister to have us so close. Each winter, there has been a crisis. The first two years, my sister's husband was very ill and Bill had to drive her to the hospital and convalescent home frequently. In addition, after two years, he needed custodial nursing care and we both helped her find a suitable nursing home. He is still alive and my sister visits him regularly."

She continued with her story. "The third year my sister had an emotional breakdown and had to be hospitalized for a number of months. It was most fortunate that we lived here because she probably made a quicker recovery due to our love and support. She is now completely well and, in turn, was available to us when we needed her this past year. Two summers ago Bill had extensive knee surgery and he took a couple of months to recover. And then, quite suddenly last winter, he required a bypass operation."

Their daughter moved to Florida two years ago. She became pregnant shortly thereafter, and had a very bad time during the pregnancy and after the birth of her child. "And this happened just when Bill had his heart surgery," Sandra said. "I didn't know which way to turn. I was running in two directions between my husband and my daughter. My sister was most supportive during these crises. She was extremely thoughtful, loving, and giving. She helped me in running errands for each of them and I don't know what I would have done without her."

Because of her family situation for the past three years, Sandra does not feel that she has had an opportunity to enjoy Florida or to make any new friends. She said, "This year, for the first time, everything is going fine. This is our first good year in Florida. I have not been able to do any real socializing because of the magnitude of our family crises. I think that I'm finally adjusting to my new home and that things are looking up and getting better."

In addition to her sister and their daughter's family, Bill has a sister and brother-in-law who spend almost four months in Florida and a cousin and her husband who spend part of the winter in Florida. Also, during the winter, many of their northern friends visit them. Sandra is now going on short trips with her sister and is enjoying being a grandmother.

Her present, more positive attitude about her living arrangement has made Sandra feel that if there are no other traumatic situations she will be free to become more active in community life. She plans to explore volunteer organizations and courses at the local university. She is interested in a group called We Care that helps homebound elderly with shopping and home-delivered meals, and a literacy group for older people. She is also planning for her husband and herself to learn to play bridge because she says, "If you don't play cards or other games, it is difficult to meet people and make new friends."

Basically, according to Sandra, they moved south because of her husband's strong desire to be outdoors every day and because she wanted to be near her sister. Her sister is older and is aging quickly and becoming quite fragile. Bill has been helping her sister with her checks, income tax, and other financial matters. She joins them for social evenings and on day or overnight trips. Bill likes and respects

Sandra's sister. Sandra said, with obvious pleasure, "He is very kind, gentle, and supportive of her and they get along extremely well."

In contrast to his wife, Bill loves to be outdoors and misses the sports activities that he can no longer do because of his damaged knee. As a young adult he had liked dancing, but since Sandra does not dance he has not danced since they were married. Also, "Unlike my wife," he said, "no culture for me—no concerts, no dance programs, no theater." He does enjoy listening to classical music tapes on his tape deck. He had no time to read outside his field while he was working but since his retirement, "I have gone back to serious reading for pleasure, mainly biographies."

Bill described his life-style while working as being all consuming, but said, "I was home a lot more than most husbands and I enjoyed spending that kind of time with my family." His attitude about leaving his home in the North was in sharp contrast to his wife's. "I hated living in a big city and had always wanted to live in a small town. I couldn't wait to leave the filth and the crime, although I was very happy teaching at the college."

He did confess that when he first visited his sister-in-law in Florida eight years ago, he was not favorably impressed and commented, "Everyone seemed so old and at the college I was used to seeing mainly young students. Also, the people seemed to be simple and uneducated and would not provide a very stimulating environment. However, when I returned a few years later I found the weather and the outdoor activities very appealing and began to feel more comfortable and at home here."

He said that Sandra did not really want to relocate but agreed to try it on a trial basis. He added, "I understand that I'm fairly typical of other older men in that the husbands adjust to living in the South much more quickly than their wives." Through her sister, they found a second-floor unit in her development that they rented for five months. Bill said, "I liked the weather and was tired of the cold in the North and my runny nose. I enjoyed having summer in the winter. And more importantly, I began to feel at home here."

According to Bill, when they made the decision to spend at least half the year in Florida they bought an inexpensive apartment in the same adult community where Sandra's sister lived. After a year or so, Bill was beginning to find that owning two homes was becoming too much of a burden and he convinced his wife to sell their house in the North and make Florida their permanent residence. They now spend eight or nine months in the South and rent a house in New England for the summer. Sandra felt that the apartment was too small and not attractively furnished, since it was bought originally to use as a second home. She wanted a more spacious unit with two bathrooms and to start from "scratch" and buy all new furniture. They have just purchased a new unit that has met their specifications and expect to move in the very near future.

Now that they have been living in Florida for a few years, Bill summed up his feelings that this was a positive move for both of them. The warm weather and the opportunity to spend so much time outdoors was first and foremost. He added, "Another attraction is the financial advantages that living in Florida offers. The cost of housing, real estate taxes, and car insurance are all much less than in the North, and eating out in restaurants is less expensive." And Sandra chimed in with the remark that "being so near my only sister and now our daughter and grandson has made this move even more acceptable for me."

-✠-

However, despite the many advantages of moving to a southern state, not everyone who relocates finds it easy to do. Pauline and Sam are a couple in their seventies who sold their home in the North, where they had lived for forty-two years and bought a three-bedroom house in Florida. Although they had spent many winters in the South and liked the climate and the outdoor activities, giving up their home of so many years was a real wrench, particularly for Pauline.

Pauline and Sam have one daughter who lives in the Midwest; they see her two or three times a year. Sam was a social worker who retired ten years ago. Pauline was in business and she continued to work for ten years after her only child was born. She then studied painting and bridge. This latter activity eventually became her all-consuming interest and she continues to play duplicate bridge at least three times a week. Sam's hobby is golf. They are both excellent swimmers and do laps daily in the pool.

They enjoy museums, theater, movies, and visiting and eating out with friends. In addition to spending winters in Florida, they have traveled extensively in Europe, the Caribbean, and the United States. Sam was particularly interested in getting away from the cold winters in the North and they began to explore Florida since it was closer than California and they knew many other snowbirds.

Pauline was reluctant at first to spend two months away from home, but after the first winter, she said, "I began to feel more comfortable and enjoyed it more. I found an excellent bridge partner and some very good bridge games here. Originally, I had preferred the Caribbean for two weeks but Sam wanted to be away for the whole winter and the Caribbean was too expensive for that length of time."

After renting the same house for five winters, they had to look for a new place since this house was sold. This meant finding and adjusting to a new rental each year. "I hated the next place the agent found for us. I hated it with a real passion," Pauline exclaimed. This pushed them into deciding to purchase their own house.

Although it was not difficult to find a suitable home, Pauline and Sam each had a different perspective on relocation. She preferred to keep their home in the North and spend up to half a year in Florida, at least for the time being, while he was adamant about making Florida his permanent residence immediately. Sam said, "Even if we could afford it, I didn't want the responsibility of owning two houses."

Pauline explained her position: "At seventy-two and seventy-four, you don't pick yourself up and make a major change and give up your friends and supports. Almost all my friends who stay in Florida are snowbirds and no one we know has moved permanently to Florida. I've lived in the same house, except during the war, and have never really moved. This move means giving up my roots since I was born in that area, married, and raised my family there!"

She also felt that perhaps it would have been better if they had bought a new house. "Everything would have been fresh and exciting. Also, it would have been easier to make friends since all the other residents would have been in the same boat." Pauline does not like the hot, humid summers and feels that they now have the same problem in reverse: now they have to find a place for the summer months where it is cool.

On the other hand, Sam's attitude was quite different. It was similar to the other couples we have met in this chapter. He said, "I wanted to move and live in a southern climate. My sister moved to California fifteen years ago, because her two sons live there. We have visited them many times and I would have preferred to settle there permanently. But Pauline objected, so living in Florida was a compromise. We had been coming to Florida for eight years and it was a familiar place by now and we had made many friends. I can also tolerate the heat better than my wife and it is not necessary for me to leave Florida in the summer."

Sam did not find it traumatic to give up his home. "I don't think that I get so attached to places. Also, I had prepared myself emotionally for this move and did not want the expense and the responsibility of two houses. I was glad to leave the North and the cold and be able to be outdoors all year round and play golf and swim. The older you get, the harder it is to be driving back and forth each year between the North and the South."

Pauline and Sam moved to Florida seven months ago and Sam really likes their new home and enjoys living in Florida. He plays golf twice a week, swims laps in the pool daily, and spends time on the beach whenever weather permits. He feels more stimulated and more active than he did in the North. He is taking courses in the local college once a week and is considering taking up bridge again.

Sam is a reader and enjoys spending time in the library perusing magazines. He is contemplating joining a community center that is being built in his area. He was also asked to serve on his condo board. "There are loads of activities for people who want to be busy all the time. But we're not people who want to be that active or that scheduled."

He summed up his feeling about his relocation: "I have no regrets. I find this a very easy and comfortable life." However, as I stated earlier, his wife has still not adjusted to the move. "I felt very secure in my old home. I feel very insecure here in Florida. I feel powerless, with no feeling of confidence in my ability to take care of myself. If anything happened to Sam I don't think I could survive here alone. This move has aged me. My message to other retirees is, 'Don't do it. Stay where you are!'"

Although Pauline's reaction to their relocation was rather extreme, it is a good idea to view moving one's permanent home with caution. Before deciding on any move, it is wise to rent first and try living in the new area for at least a part of the year. If it is economically feasible, one should not sell the former home until absolutely sure about living in the new house. It is important to evaluate to what extent you would miss family and friends, and how lonely you would be in the new place. If you can bring some of your furniture with you this would help in creating a feeling of familiarity and security in your new home.

Before moving to a new area, you should explore the taxes, cost of food and housing, types of facilities and services available, and the cultural, educational, volunteer, and recreational opportunities. All the couples who were interviewed here offered similar reasons for choosing to relocate. Most wanted to avoid the cold winter season and wanted a warm climate all year round. For some this was important because it offered them the opportunity to engage in outdoor activities and for others a warm climate was necessary for health reasons. Second, the relocatees wanted the easier life-style that the South offered. Third, some moved to be closer to children or other family members. And fourth, housing and taxes cost less in the South than in the North. (This is particularly true for Florida and parts of North Carolina, but may not be as true for California or Arizona.)

Dr. Charles F. Longino, Jr., has analyzed the 1980 census data for migration patterns of the elderly. His research indicated that some of the elderly who had relocated to the South and Southwest have returned home to be near children or other family when they have lost a spouse, become quite frail, or became unable to care for themselves. The people moving back from Florida tended to be older, poorer, and widowed than the group that had originally migrated to the South. They tended to move back to their former states when they could no longer manage to live independently and needed the support of adult children or other younger family members.[2]

However, the majority of those who have chosen to live in a warm climate did make a new life for themselves and remained in their new homes.

Time for a Change

Housing Alternatives for Elderly
Who Want to Move

In previous chapters I discussed ways that older people can make their homes more financially affordable and physically safer, and how they can make their lives more emotionally secure.[1] In addition, I presented the many resources and services in the community that can help the elderly remain in their own homes. Unfortunately, even with these in-home adjustments, a time may come when staying in one's own home becomes a foolish course of action. Sometimes older people gradually become weaker and more fragile or develop chronic ailments or handicaps that gradually incapacitate them. Over a period of time they become less and less able to manage the daily routines of housekeeping. Or a sudden trauma, such as a stroke or serious accident, may immediately cause such a change that the elderly person becomes incapable of living alone.

Continuing Care Retirement Communities

One such couple, Amy and Jack, found themselves in just such a position. Fourteen years ago, when Jack was seventy years old, he was forced to retire. This couple was childless and had no other family to keep them in the area, so they were free to leave the northern city where they had lived most of their lives. Jack said, "Our section of the city had deteriorated and moving to a better area would have been too costly. In addition, all the cultural events we enjoyed were becoming too expensive when you figured out the price of the tickets, parking fees, and eating in restaurants. We also began to feel less and less comfortable going out at night in the city."

They decided to move to Florida because many of their friends had already done so and because they knew they could afford to buy a condominium apartment there. They enjoyed playing golf and looked forward to being able to play all year round. Amy added, "We found many cultural activities, like concerts, theater, and dance that were much less expensive than up North. You know, Florida is not the cultural desert that many northern urban people think it is. We also found that these programs were very accessible. And college-level courses for seniors were very conveniently located."

They liked living in their Florida condominium, a two-bedroom, two-bath apartment that overlooked the golf course. In addition to renewing friendships with many old friends who had preceded them in moving to Florida, they made many new friends. An unexpected benefit of their relocation was that the condominium complex offered them opportunities for leadership roles. Amy stated, "I introduced 'Great Decisions' and 'Great Books.' Both these groups have become very popular and are still ongoing activities at the clubhouse. And my husband gave a series of five or six lectures yearly on chamber music. We had over two hundred people attending, many of whom had never heard any chamber music before."

Jack chimed in with, "And don't forget what we both did in the men's and women's clubs."

"That's right. When we first joined these groups, they focused mainly on discussing condo affairs. But we introduced the idea that we should act more like a public forum and action group and should be involved in local, state, and national issues," Amy said.

The only negative thing about life in Florida was summer: "The weather here in the summer is intolerable," Jack stated. They spend six weeks each summer in the western part of New York State attending a cultural institute.

But after eleven years of living independently in their condominium they began to look to the future. Now Jack was eighty-one and Amy seventy-nine. Jack explained his feelings at this point in his life: "I was scared. Who would take care of us if one of us became very ill or died? I was beginning to feel quite insecure living by ourselves. The high cost of nursing care has bankrupted even wealthy people. So Amy and I decided to do some reading about housing alternatives for older people and began to visit some of them in the area."

After exploring the subject quite thoroughly, they decided that a life-care community (LCC), or, as they now are called, a continuing care retirement community (CCRC), would answer their needs. This type of housing provides the benefits associated with having an independent apartment but also offers meals, linen service, housekeeping, medical services (except for acute care in a hospital), and a nursing home.

Amy and Jack were fortunate to find a CCRC that they could afford in the same neighborhood where they had been living. Amy said, "Because of this we were able to retain our ties to our cultural activities and our friends from the condo."

Jack said, "It is important to pick a place where the residents are compatible with you. Unfortunately, that isn't as true here and is one of the errors that we made in choosing this place. But we like everything else about it. We like the fact that we have a contract which states that we will be cared for our entire lives, no matter what our health conditions are. We have a very highly rated health center which makes me feel very secure."

Amy offered, "I love our large and attractive apartment. It's a wonderful way to live as you get older. It relieves me of my house-hold cares like housekeeping, semiannual cleaning, and heavy food shopping. It's also a good place for people who can no longer drive since our place offers transportation to shopping malls and medical and hospital appointments."

In the two years they have lived in the life-care facility, the support services and the residents' caring has been of great help to them, particularly during Jack's recent illness. He required a major operation that necessitated several weeks in the hospital and an additional month in a rehabilitation center. He is now at home and is receiving help from the in-house medical staff. Their present living arrangement made it much easier for them to survive this difficult period.

Amy said, "I don't know how I would have managed if not for the meals program and the help of some of the residents. I have a vision problem which makes it impossible for me to drive at night. During this six-week period when Jack was hospitalized, several of the men insisted on taking me to visit my husband most evenings. It was so important for me to see him and helped him get well more quickly. I was able to eat a regular dinner each evening in the company of caring people, which kept me on an even keel, physically and emotionally. And you know, in addition to our old friends' support, Jack received over a hundred notes and get-well cards from the residents."

Of all the housing alternatives for the elderly, life-care communities (LCC) or continuing care retirement communities (CCRC) are the first choice of middle- and upper-income elderly. These people enjoy the comfort of knowing that no matter what the state of their health, they will be cared for throughout their lives. The contractual agreement between each resident and the CCRC guarantees health care until the end of the resident's life, except during hospital stays. An entry fee paid at the time of acceptance into the facility covers all the stages of care that the resident may need in the future. CCRCs have nursing homes directly on their grounds. Thus, if a resident needs either short- or long-term nursing care, the elderly person can receive needed attention while staying in close touch with friends in the community. For married couples, the proximity of a nursing home can be a special blessing, because it makes daily visiting easier and can make it seem as if the husband and wife are still living together.

The apartments in a CCRC may be in a new high-rise, a mid-rise, or a low, campus-style building, or in a renovated, older building such as a hotel-motel, school, or office complex. Each individual or couple has a separate self-contained unit, ranging in size from a studio apartment with sleeping area to a one- or two-bedroom apartment, plus bath, small kitchen, and living-dining room. Communal spaces are provided for dining, social, recreational, and hobby activities.

In addition to a high entry fee, a resident pays a monthly fee for apartment rental. This fee also covers the cost of at least one meal a day, housekeeping and linen services, recreational and cultural programs, transportation, and twenty-four-hour medical emergency service.

Ridgecrest Retirement Residence, a CCRC located on the edge of the town where Linda lived, was operated by a church-sponsored nonprofit corporation. The community consisted of attractive one- and two-bedroom cluster cottages and two lodge-type buildings that each contained a dozen studio units. On the grounds a large, barnlike structure served as dining room and meeting hall. A two-story brick building housed health-related and skilled nursing facilities. The entry fee for admittance to Ridgecrest was substantial because of the expenses involved in maintaining good residential and nursing facilities. Despite the cost, Linda urged her mother, Susan, who had a severe heart attack and continued to suffer from fainting spells that frequently sent her to the hospital, to make out an application for Ridgecrest.

"It wasn't easy getting mother to fill out the form. She insisted she never wanted to move again," Linda recalled. Her mom had moved from her large suburban house in the Northwest to a nearby city apartment after her husband's—Linda's father's—death. "But I told her there was a four-year waiting period and that she wouldn't be obligated to accept an apartment if and when one became available. It was like insurance."

Her mother's resistance to living in a CCRC broke down after her best friend died. Her fainting spells increased and she seemed to lose the will to live. By the time Susan moved into a one-bedroom cottage unit that became available at Ridgecrest, she no longer cared about either where or even whether she lived. As Susan looked back on that period more than a year later, she remembered, "I could accept the move intellectually, but not emotionally. I didn't make any effort to be friendly or to join in any activities. If it were up to me I'd have stayed in the cottage all day. But management insists you come to the dining room for dinner every evening. And Linda came almost every day and dragged me out—to play bridge, to go to special luncheons and meetings. Now I belong to a regular bridge group. And I've joined a few committees and found some friends I really feel comfortable with."

As Susan joined a book discussion group, the county art society, the residents' trip-planning committee, and volunteered for desk work at the town's birth-control clinic, her general health improved. Now she says, "I do think this is a lovely place. And I guess I can truthfully say, that, at last, I feel at home here."

-✼-

For the Hales, the decision to move into a CCRC in Pennsylvania came after her husband and then she herself decided to give up driving.[1] This meant that they would have to look into a life-style arrangement that did not depend on the use of a car.

As Mrs. Hale wrote, choosing a CCRC "proved to be the wisest decision we ever made. We found a place where all our needs were met—a spacious apartment with a view, proximity to a fine hospital, nourishing meals attractively served, twenty-four-hour security, transportation for shopping, and friendly, congenial people.

Although the entrance and monthly fees seemed steep, the Hales "were pleased to learn that the IRS allows a generous percentage of the monthly fee and the entrance fee as a medical deduction." When it became necessary for her husband to have nursing care, Mrs. Hale felt that "he received more loving care there [at the medical center] than he would have received at the usual nursing home." Daily visits were easier, too, because the nursing facility was on the grounds of the CCRC.

To conclude Mrs. Hale's story in her own words: "When my husband died, I was fortunate to have the support of warm friends. Because many of them have known the pain of bereavement, they were able to help me greatly during a very sad time. At eighty-nine, I walk about a mile a day, using a cane as a safety measure. The days are never long enough to accomplish all I plan, but each day I give thanks for having found a beautiful place to live and good friends to share it with."

Congregate Residences

If one cannot afford a CCRC or does not want a medically oriented community, a congregate residence is another option. Feld House, a fifteen-story building with 250 studio and one-bedroom apartments, is one of the oldest senior citizens' housing complexes in the United States; it was started over 30 years ago. The minimum age for admittance is 62. No entrance fee is charged, and the monthly fee, though substantially less than in a CCRC, pays for the rent of an apartment, two meals daily (lunch and dinner), housekeeping, plus a variety of social, recreational, and cultural programs.

Feld House is located in a mixed working- and middle-class neighborhood with stores, a bank, and a luncheonette near at hand. Residents from the building who wish to be actively involved in the neighborhood can discuss politics on the park benches two blocks away in good weather or work as volunteers at a hospital and social service agency in the vicinity.

In the mornings most residents prepare their own breakfasts in the small kitchens of their apartments. Residents who are disoriented or seriously impaired are not allowed to have working stoves, so they eat in the main dining room between 8:00 and 9:30 A.M. Other residents occasionally join them, especially for the Sunday pancake breakfasts, at a small extra cost.

Perhaps one-fourth of the residents were out of the building at lunchtime on days when the weather was good. At one time they had tried to convince the management that the midday meal as well as breakfast should be optional. But an emphasis on good nutrition at Feld House made the management reluctant to leave the responsibility of eating a well-balanced lunch to the vagaries of the residents. Dora, who was eighty-one and had lived in the senior citizens' complex for five years, had been an original agitator for the change at lunchtime. But she too admits rather grudgingly that the older people she knows have a tendency to eat little for breakfast, and that they might skimp again at lunch or even forget to eat lunch if left to make the decision themselves.

Getting used to the regime of eating meals every day at the same time had been difficult for Dora. But her daughter saw the soundness of the policy, since she knew that Dora had been careless about eating properly when she had lived at home alone.

In her first years at Feld House, Dora volunteered as a teacher's aide at a neighborhood elementary school. Increasing distress from her arthritic condition forced her to give up that activity. But she still continues to involve herself in neighborhood affairs—arguing politics and staunchly defending the rights of the underdog.

In addition, she has added several new interests to occupy her: painting and choral singing. Both these hobbies can be pursued in the building. On the lower level is a large studio with easels and work tables. An adjacent room contains long tables with colorful yarns, a few needlepoint frames, and exotic birds and flowers that residents had made from brightly colored crepe paper. Beyond the crafts area and the laundry room is an auditorium with a piano on one side and a small stage where concerts are held and the choir meets for practice. The large auditorium is also used for meetings, parties, and movies.

Dora admitted that she would never have had the energy to explore stimulating new hobbies and friendships if she had to struggle each day with keeping house and preparing meals for herself. The discovery of these activities and the forming of new friendships gives her the impetus to get going each morning. "No matter how stiff and creaky I feel, I'm glad to get up every morning," she explained.

Like most residents at Feld House, Dora wakes at the first sign of light. "I hug my pillow until my mind frees itself from the cobwebs. Then I think about my plans for the day until the juices start flowing." After a warm shower, she prepares breakfast. She is glad that this meal was not part of the service package, because she feels that old people need to go at their own pace in the morning. After breakfast, she makes her bed, tidies her rooms, and heads for the elevator. On the way she raps on one of the doors with her cane. A woman calls from inside, "Is that you, Dora?" An affirmative answer brings her to the door.

"How are you this morning, Bessie?" Dora asked.

"I think I'll live the day."

"Good!" Dora said cheerily.

By 8:30 A.M. the lounge downstairs at Feld House is a beehive of activity. Dora is joined by Bessie and another woman. They hold an earnest discussion about what they would do that day. After art class and lunch, they would shop for stockings at the discount store near the bank. That settled, they comment on what is happening in the world as they read their newspapers.

Dora's determination and her adaptability made it fairly easy for her to make the transition to the life-style of congregate housing. Not everyone adjusts as smoothly, her daughter Shirley recalls. "I've realized for a long time how wise Mom was to move to Feld while she still had the energy and health to enjoy the activities."

Shirley described Dora as a "superefficient housekeeper." After she fell and broke her right hip, she began to have problems with housekeeping and shopping. She saw Feld House when a friend moved there and right away, without discussing her decision with her daughter or her two sons, she put in her application. "It wouldn't be too easy for her now, her arthritis has gotten so bad."

Shirley recognized now that her mother had acted in a sensible and self-reliant way, although back then she had felt bad about her mother's decision. She had felt that her childhood home was being abandoned and that her mother was not ready for an "institution." Yet it had been a good thing Dora made the decision when she did.

Shirley explained that since her mother's move to Feld House she and her brothers had had the assurance that their mother was safe and eating well, seeing her doctor, and taking her medication. Shirley admitted that if her mother had tried to stick it out alone in her apartment it would have meant a lot of work and a lot of worry for her and her brothers.

Knowing when to make the change is critical. Dora's sister, Mary, had stayed in her own apartment too long, depending on her children to clean, shop, and care for her. By the time she made the change to Feld House at the age of 88, it was too late. She had become too despondent and infirm to take part in the activities and to form the friendships that are such an important part of life for the elderly who live successful and productive lives.

Government-Subsidized Housing for the Elderly

Although congregate housing is less costly than a CCRC, both options are far too expensive for the low- or moderate-income older person with limited or no assets or savings. A housing option for such elderly people is securing an apartment in a government-subsidized project for senior citizens.

I visited a typical example of subsidized housing located in a small midwestern city. Avery Square Apartments consists of four three-story buildings built around an open court with a small park in its center. Ninety-eight elderly tenants live in eighty-five apartments. With the aid of a state grant, congregate services are offered to a small percentage of the tenants; they receive one cooked meal a day, housekeeping services, and personal care—help with such things as bathing, dressing, shopping, and care of clothing.

Elinor, eighty-six years old, could not have managed to stay in her apartment without the aid of household help and meals. Leaning heavily on her walker, she showed me around her apartment: a small kitchen and bedroom; a windowless bathroom with grab bars, stall shower, and emergency buzzer cord; and an average-sized living room with two windows overlooking the courtyard. Nine years ago when she moved in, Elinor could still manage shopping and cooking by herself, but after five years, she needed extra help. "I don't know what I'd do," Elinor said. "I just know I'd never want to move in with any of my children or friends."

By her "children," Elinor, a former teacher and administrator who had never married, meant her students. She had kept in touch with quite a few, and two who took a special interest in her she regarded as her sons. Although no legal adoption had taken place, these boys, who had been in the children's home where she taught, were her family. "My boys offered to help out. And I had friends who wanted me to come and live with them. But I preferred to live independently, as I always have," Elinor stated.

In general, Elinor liked life at Avery Square. She led a busy life. She served on the tenants' council, frequently went on trips planned by and for the seniors, and played bingo in the afternoons. She also made a point of walking twice around the park on days when she did not walk the two blocks to the neighborhood shopping center. Considering that all her movements were very laborious, these walks—often taken with a blind neighbor, since walking together helped each to keep up their resolve—were feats of great courage.

-¤-

Avery Square was also home to eighty-three-year-old Diana, who had come from Yorkshire, England, after her husband's death, to live with her only child, Edwina, who was married to an American college professor. Edwina recalled her mother's condition then: "When my dad died, everything was shattered. Mum depended on him for everything. There wasn't much money. He'd only been a state-school teacher, and she'd earned a little giving piano lessons. And the old house was falling down 'round their ears. Both getting on in years, you know. Then Dad's being so ill and all. It really sent Mum into an awful state of depression."

For four years Diana had lived in Edwina's home without much sign of improvement in her despondency. "It really is not good for the old to live with the young," Diana commented. "I felt very strongly that I should have a place of my own. I wanted to be near Edwina and the family, of course, but I didn't want to live in their house."

Avery Square Apartments proved to be the perfect solution: only a few miles from the house where Edwina and her husband had lived for almost thirty years, it was ideal in terms of location, set-up, and costs. Although there was a two-year waiting list, they were patient.

A short time after Diana moved in, Edwina quickly began to notice a change in her mother. Diana started to play the piano in Edwina's living room again; later she performed for the other residents in the community room and then accepted the job of accompanist at church choir rehearsals. Her social life brightened as she began to make new friends, inviting them to lunch or afternoon tea or going to their apartments when they reciprocated. "I can scarcely believe my eyes sometimes. Is this the same sad lady who moped around my house? It's really quite wonderful how her real spirit and lively nature have returned since she moved to Avery Square," Edwina exclaimed.

It was comforting, too, to know that although Diana did not yet require congregate services, she could apply for them in the future. Unfortunately, government-subsidized housing that provides congregate services is an exception rather than the rule. The majority of residents living in subsidized housing for the elderly have to make do without these support services. They rely on younger family members or neighbors, or turn to community social agencies for needed services, or they may be forced to find other more semidependent living arrangements.

In order to qualify for a federal- or state-subsidized housing unit, one must be sixty-two years old or older, fall within specified income guidelines, and be able to care for oneself. Those accepted pay only 30 percent of their income for rent. Unfortunately, in many parts of the country, government-subsidized elderly housing projects have long waiting lists. Despite the need, new construction has been sharply curtailed since the early 1980s.

Group-Shared Homes

CCRCs, congregate housing, and government-subsidized projects are usually large building complexes, with one hundred to four hundred apartment units. But many elderly prefer a smaller, more homelike atmosphere. For these seniors there is an option called group-shared homes.

Edna was widowed just after her thirty-fourth wedding anniversary. Disaster struck on the family suddenly with no previous warning. Only fifty-eight, Edna adjusted relatively well to the loss. She missed her husband, but she made new friends and became active in organizations that were interested in improving the local schools and in protecting the environment. With her daughter Carol, Edna attended zoning board and town planning board meetings. She became president of the local chapter of the League of Women Voters and a few years later won a seat on the school district's board of education. Her life was busy: she took courses is psychology and languages at a nearby college, and played tennis and bridge regularly.

But in her early seventies, Edna developed cataracts. Despite several operations, she suffered a loss of vision that led to a curtailment of many of her activities. Unable to drive, she resisted calling others to give her a lift to meetings. She began to spend more time alone in her apartment. For someone who enjoyed people and involvement, the solitude was very destructive. And then a bout with pneumonia led to a long and slow convalescence spent partially at Carol's house. It was at this point that Edna said, "I definitely don't want to make this my permanent home. My mother lived with me for most of my married life and she lived to be ninety-three. I won't do that to my daughter."

She was not ready for a nursing home, Edna observed, but on the other hand, she did not have enough energy for Sun City. Carol mentioned the possibility of living in some sort of retirement residence or adult home and Edna snorted, "Old-age homes, you mean." Faced with this impasse, Carol told her mother that if she were her old self, she would not be thinking that way. With all the community projects she had tackled and the battles she had fought for others, she had no right giving up on herself.

Edna needed that encouragement. "Thanks, Honey, I needed to be reminded that I am a person of worth. When you feel inadequate and useless, you tend to forget all your old strengths."

Once they settled on the advisability of investigating housing options, the pair proceeded as though they were conducting a committee study for one of their organizations. Edna telephoned several area agencies on aging and asked for lists of residences and housing programs. Carol contacted the state housing finance agency and the county community development department and obtained information on new and proposed projects. Together they looked into traditional housing for the elderly, as well as innovative concepts in shared and cooperative living.

After several months of exploring different housing options, Edna decided that a group-shared home fit her pocketbook and suited her life-style. This type of living arrangement has begun to sprout up around the country in the past ten years. In a group-shared home, at least five, but as many as fifteen, unrelated people agree to live together and share the expenses and part or even all of the work involved in keeping up the household. The concept may sound like the communes of the 1960s. In communes people lived together so that they could enjoy the economic advantages that come from pooling their resources, as well as a sense of community or family. Often people entered communes to find security and to escape chaos in their lives. A group-shared home serves the same purpose: it allows older people to live more economically, provides companionship, and offers a protected place where there are others close at hand to turn to when help is needed.

While the communes of the 1960s were formed by private groups who banded together, most elderly group-shared homes are sponsored by community organizations, such as churches, civic associations, advocacy groups, and government agencies. Most elderly people do not have the stamina to organize such households; they would have to plan well in advance while they were still in command of the physical energy required to set up this complex kind of living arrangement.

Group-shared homes operate with varying degrees of independence. In some the residents themselves do all the chores: cooking, cleaning, shopping, and light maintenance. At the other end of the scale are homes that have full-time, live-in housekeeping managers and staff. At the midpoint are residences where paid staff or volunteers help with some meal preparations, household tasks, and social needs.

Parkside is a large, three-story house, built in the 1930s, situated in a medium-sized town in a mid-Atlantic state. This group-shared home accommodates seven older adults: five women and two men. Each of the residents has a private bedroom and shares a bathroom with one other person.

A resident housekeeper lives in a small apartment on the third floor. The paid live-in housekeeper does the marketing, prepares dinner with the assistance of two rotating residents who are the day's kitchen helpers, keeps records of costs, cleans the common rooms and baths, and changes the linens weekly. She is around in case an emergency arises and she mediates arguments among the residents.

Near the front entryway on the first floor of the house is a small sitting area. At the end of the hallway is a large living room furnished cheerfully with a flowery, chintz-covered couch, two well-stuffed armchairs, a large television set, and a highly polished Queen Anne table. At the far end of the living room an opening leads to a large dining room. The kitchen, which had been completely modernized and is sparkling clean, has a pass-through counter and wide entry into the dining room.

Upstairs the bedrooms are furnished with possessions that had formerly been in the occupants' homes. Some furnishings and accessories in the common rooms also came from the residents, but most had been donated or bought with funds donated by the community and the sponsoring church congregation.

Parkside came into existence through the efforts of a church committee when several members of the congregation joined together because they had elderly parents who were living alone. Some of the parents lived in distant states and all of them had health problems. It appeared to the members of the church committee that the most practical project they could undertake was the establishment of a small group home. The concept was appealing because it would provide an economical, dignified, caring atmosphere for their parents who should or could no longer live alone and who did not want to make a permanent home with their children.

Turning the concept into a reality was a lot of work for a lot of people. "So many permits, licenses, approvals, and what-alls to get. And all from different agencies of the town, county, and state. Seemed like there were hundreds of them." This observation was made by Virginia, who at seventy-two was the youngest resident of the group-shared home. She described the planning and work that went into remodeling the house. An architect worked with the property committee to ascertain the changes that were needed and then drew up a set of blueprints without charging a fee. The housing corporation, formed to develop and manage the project, served as general contractor; the church building committee obtained bids, let contracts, and checked on the work's progress.

Virginia was part of the team that showed up every day to push the construction along. She explained that that task and cleaning up were the hard parts. The fun part was the interior painting and decorating that was done by volunteers with everyone pitching in, including children and grandchildren. At that time, she was certainly not thinking about moving into Parkside. She and her husband lived about a mile away from the project in a pleasant cottage that had been their home for most of the forty-eight years of their marriage. But a few months after the group-shared home opened, Virginia's husband suddenly died, and she felt as though the ground fell away. Having never lived alone, every sound was magnified and she was terrified being by herself at night.

Virginia's son suggested that she give Parkside a try. He proposed that she rent her house for a year and if she changed her mind, she could come back to it. "I don't think I want to go back, but I have a few months to make up my mind. One thing is sure," Virginia added, "I don't want to leave this town, and this location is wonderful. My church is around the corner, and I like being close enough to walk to the library, bank, and stores that I'm used to."

-⚹-

At eighty-eight, Christa is the oldest resident at Parkside. She came there from a nursing home, where she had gone after a hospital stay for a broken shoulder and arm suffered in a fall on her bathroom floor. Her son refused to let her return to her apartment and made the arrangements to move her to Parkside. Christa accepted them with some misgivings.

Widowed for twenty years, Christa had been an assistant principal at a large city high school. After her retirement, she took a year's tour with a woman friend around the country in a large camper, and lived in New Mexico with a man, a college friend whom she met again on her travels. She stayed with him until the relationship soured and then she headed east again and moved into a city apartment, so that she could attend concerts and the theater.

Restless and spunky, Christa did not spend much time chatting with the other women in the home, but she had developed a special, caring relationship with Jim, one of the male residents, who was more than ten years her junior. He looked after her, helping her up the stairs to her second-floor bedroom or making her a cup of tea when she wandered into the kitchen at dawn, bleary-eyed because she had had trouble sleeping.

Both Jim and Christa were important to one another. Jim had come to the home after a suicide attempt, following the death of his wife, whom he had devotedly nursed through a long-term illness. Parkside was a retreat for him: he was handy at fixing things and at taking care of the garden and mowing the lawn.

The group-shared home formed a supportive environment for the others too. Three of the women, Virginia, Belle, and Jean, had become close companions. They almost always had breakfast together, and lunch too, if they were not out somewhere. The newest residents, Bill and Rose, had been at Parkside for only a few months. They were still in the settling-in stage, a period of adjustment that varies with individual residents.

Mabel, the residents' committee chairwoman, a social worker in her early forties, gave me further insights into the nature of the home and its tenants. "The people aren't really a family; they have no common history to bind them together," Mabel remarked. "The need for companionship, security, and housekeeping help at a reasonable cost is what brought them here," Mabel continued in her forthright manner. "They know they can stay for as long as their health and strength hold out. Best of all, they have as much independence as they can handle without the loneliness and insecurity of living alone or the guilt of being a burden on their children."

Parkside's setting in a converted, old, single-family house in a suburban town might be a difficult adjustment for a city person. On the other hand, Valdene's location might be just the thing for a confirmed urban dweller. Valdene, a group-shared home composed of a cluster of five three-bedroom apartments in a twenty-two-story building, was set up in a high-rise apartment building in a middle-class neighborhood in a northeastern city. The apartments are rented and supervised by a community service agency.

The project opened in 1979 with room for twelve residents in four apartments. The landlord gave permission to remove the walls between two adjacent apartments, thus creating a large communal space for serving the main meal each day and for resident meetings and parties.

A resident manager, who lives in a separate apartment in the building, is responsible for the marketing and cooking. The manager has the help of two part-time assistants. The manager also supervises the cleaning staff and is on round-the-clock call. A social worker-counselor spends 15 hours each week with residents, discussing problems ranging from personal feelings of insecurity and health complaints to personality clashes among apartment mates.

In the apartment shared by Lila, in her ninety-second year, and two octogenarians, Jenny and Rachel, there existed the usual mix of harmony and discord one might expect to find when diverse people live in close quarters. Lila, partially deaf and almost blind, had suffered a major heart attack. She had been living in the group-shared residence for five years and every day was exciting for her. She attended a senior day-care program, and was driven back and forth in the Valdene van. Jenny, eighty-five, had crippling arthritis that forced her to use a cane or hold the kitchen countertops as she moved awkwardly around the room. Modest and proud, Jenny had been upset at first at the thought of having to ask a perfect stranger to help her zip up her dress. "But you soon learn that living together, you don't stay strangers for very long," she explained.

The third apartment mate, Rachel, eighty-six, was a former schoolteacher. She had had a series of small strokes after her husband's death and sometimes used a walker when she felt shaky. She made the following assessment of Valdene: "Life here isn't bad, but it's not a bed of roses. We're all set in our ways, and we get on each other's nerves sometimes. One plays her TV too loud. One clomps around the kitchen at night when she can't sleep. One leaves crumbs all over the living room."

"On the other hand," she continued, "it's good to know there's someone here to talk to and if you get sick suddenly, you feel a lot safer. And it takes the strain off your children."

All the apartments at Valdene are occupied by women. Three men had never made applications at the same time. Roslyn, the manager of Valdene, explained that there was a reluctance about having men and women sharing the same apartment. Half the women who lived at Valdene chose it themselves; the other half were persuaded to try it by their children. The biggest problem, according to Roslyn, was that by the time an applicant and her family were ready to accept group living, the older person might be too frail or too impaired to be able to cope with this type of living arrangement.

Group-shared homes are for people who have certain economic, physical, or emotional problems that make it difficult or impossible for them to live alone. It is this common bond that draws them together. For the majority, living with their children is not a viable solution. They want to live close enough to their families to enjoy regular visits and family support in the event of serious illness. But basically they wish to remain independent.

Of course, it is obvious that group-sharing participants must have a decent level of tolerance for the foibles of their apartment mates, as well as sufficient flexibility to trade some privacy for companionship, care, and financial advantages. Most older people would not be able to manage the adjustment without continued attention from family members. Without family support, the older person might feel bitter and abandoned. Most children understand this need, and actually have a better relationship once the burden, the anxieties, and the uncertainties of caring for an elderly parent are lessened.

Group-shared homes all have the same purpose: they extend the years of independence for the elderly person who has become too frail or impaired to continue living alone. And, of course, the community benefits too by reducing pressure on more costly community resources such as nursing homes, hospitals, and social service agencies.

Adult Communities

In the last chapter we met couples who had moved to Florida, most of whom were living in an adult community, another housing option. These communities are complexes of permanent dwelling units for older adults, where the minimum age requirements for members range from forty-eight to fifty-five. These communities usually require at least one occupant to be the minimum age or older and ban children under the age of eighteen from permanent residence. They range in size from as few as one hundred units to as many as forty-five thousand, with the average falling into the four to five thousand range. Most of the adult communities are concentrated in Arizona, California, Florida, Texas, and New Jersey.

Almost always located far from town centers on tracts of undeveloped land available at low cost, large adult communities can grow into self-contained towns. Most have community centers, clubhouses, and a variety of sports and recreational facilities; some have their own shopping centers; a few even have health-care facilities.

A comfortable retirement income is needed to pay the purchase price of a condominium unit and the monthly fees for recreation and maintenance services. All communities provide some maintenance service, although this practice varies widely: some provide service only for the grounds, exterior repairs, and dwelling-unit upkeep; others provide water and sewage facilities, security police, street cleaning, interior repairs, painting, and so on. Bus or van transportation may also be provided.

Essentially, adult communities create a carefree, secure, clean, well-ordered environment for friendly, outgoing, physically active older adults who are in relatively good health—people who feel they have "paid their dues" to family and society and now want to enjoy life or play in the sun.

Mobile-Home Parks

Another of today's retirement options is the mobile-home park. The greatest concentration of such parks is in the western and southern states, but they can be found throughout the country. Most mobile-home parks are not age-specific, but many are age-dense, that is, they house large numbers of residents who are 60 and older. Buying a mobile home and paying low monthly fees to keep it in a mobile-home park is far less expensive than buying a home in an adult condominium community or paying for congregate housing or for entry into a CCRC. Many parks have clubhouses, but group activities are usually generated and organized by the residents themselves.

Residential Hotels

Some of the elderly, dissatisfied with living alone, choose to move into residential hotels. "Residential hotel" is a broad term used to cover a wide range of accommodations, from modest to luxurious. Those specifically designed for the elderly are called retirement hotels, some of which may have planned recreation and leisure activities. Furnished rooms, maid and linen service, and two or three meals a day are provided at costs that approximate congregate housing fees. Most residential hotels are run as private, for-profit enterprises, whereas most congregate residences are under nonprofit church-related ownership. Residential hotel living, probably because it is less structured, is also less cohesive and less conducive to making friends and developing mutual aid and support than some of the other communal living arrangements.

Board-and-Care Homes

For the older person who is having difficulty coping with daily life in the home and who needs more supervision than is given in other living arrangements, a board-and-care home may be the answer. Once a fixture in every town, providing housing for young bachelors, spinsters, widows and widowers, today boarding homes have almost disappeared. Those that survive tend to be used to house the frail and the mentally and emotionally impaired patients released from institutions. They often shelter and care for people of mixed ages, many of whom have not lived in their own homes for a long time. Coming from dependent environments, boarding home residents are less able to cope with life's challenges and require more supervision than congregate housing or group-shared living residents.

In general concept, board-and-care homes are similar to group-shared homes, but the former are usually larger—housing twenty-five to thirty residents—as compared with the five to fifteen in most group homes. A smaller size and less regulation in group-shared homes enable residents to have greater control over their own lives and create a better climate for formation of a substitute-family atmosphere.

A foster home is another possible alternative for the more dependent older person. It differs from a board-and-care home in that it is a single-family household with no more than four nonrelatives living in as paying guests. A good foster home will treat residents as family members, encouraging them to participate in normal family activities.

Board-and-care foster homes are licensed and strictly regulated in many states. Their elderly residents often have little income, receiving only supplemental security income from the Social Security Administration, so there is little financial incentive for those seeking profits to operate these types of homes. In order to keep them up to standards, some state governments have funding programs that offer assistance. Increasing shortages of affordable supportive housing for the elderly and the high cost of nursing homes may engender more support for board-and-care and foster homes in the future.

Portable Housing

One innovative way to allow elderly relatives to enjoy private but supportive housing is Elder Cottage Housing Opportunity (ECHO) housing. An elder cottage is a compact, free-standing, self-contained housing unit that can be set up adjacent to a single-family home. In Australia, where they are called "granny flats," more than five hundred are in use. The Victoria Ministry of Housing installs and rents the cottages, which are moved from place to place as needed.

Efficiency units can be as small as three hundred square feet, one- and two-bedroom units as large as nine hundred square feet. They are produced at a factory and can be finished in a variety of exterior designs to match the design of the main house on the site. In most cases, the cottages can be put up in one day, including electrical, water, and sewer hook-ups, and can be disassembled in the same amount of time.

In essence, ECHO housing is property sharing rather than house sharing, but it offers the same benefits—economy, independence, support, security, and companionship—with more privacy for elderly people and supportive families than any other sharing arrangement. The drawback is that zoning codes and public attitudes have severely limited the use of ECHO housing in this country. Although the idea has been floating around for many years and has attracted wide attention, only a few localities have passed permissive legislation and few cottages have been installed so far.

A rural county in one eastern state has started a demonstration program using three elder cottages. Each cottage contains a bedroom, living room, dining area, kitchen, and bath. Purchase price and installation costs total about $20,000. The county retains ownership of the cottages, and tenants pay a monthly rental fee that can be as low as $250. The rent is used to cover the cost of installation, insurance, and maintenance and to create a fund for the purchase of additional units in the future. When the cottage is no longer needed in one location, the county will move it to another.

Funding for the purchase of the first three units and to run the program came from state and federal housing funds. Income ceilings were set for occupants, who were limited to two people per cottage. At least one occupant had to be sixty years of age or older and related by blood, marriage, or adoption to at least one person living in the permanent residence. Other regulations specified that the owner must live on the property and set requirements concerning space and access to utility lines. Special-use permits were obtained from the municipalities where cottages were to be located.

Most applicants, according to the program director, were widows in their seventies, frail but still able to manage, who wanted to remain close to or move closer to children. The children signaled their consent by registering as joint applicants. Margaret, a seventy-six-year-old widow with a limited income and arthritic legs, was a typical candidate. For several years after her husband died she had rented the upstairs apartment in a two-family house. But the stairs became too difficult for her to negotiate and she had to leave, giving away or selling most of her furniture. After that, Margaret lived with her son's family in a small house in town for three months, then moved to her daughter's place outside of town for the next three months, before moving back with her son for another three months. She had signed up for an apartment in a senior housing project, but there was a waiting list of several years; in addition, the project was more than thirty miles from her hometown and family.

"The cottage has been a godsend," said Margaret's daughter, Bridget. "Ma's close enough so that we can keep an eye on her. Yet she can putter around all on her own without getting underfoot in my house, which isn't very large, as you can see." Bridget and her husband were coapplicants for the cottage because their house stood on a one-acre lot, whereas her brother's house in town had little acreage around it.

"My mother is a simple woman," Bridget said. "She's never done any other job than being a housewife and a mother. She never even learned to drive. She's always depended on someone else for transportation—first my dad, now me and my brother. Anyway, I can't tell you how much it means to have her nearby, safe and sound in my backyard."

The cottage, about twenty feet behind the house, could not be seen from the front yard. A miniature house complete with white plastic siding and black asphalt roof, it resembled the main house but was much newer and brighter. Margaret welcomed me inside cheerfully. The aroma of cinnamon and ginger filled the neat little house, so it was no surprise when my hostess, a woman of medium height, large girth, and hobbling movements, told me she had just baked some cookies and offered me a cup of tea.

The interior was much like a motel unit, with imitation wood paneling on the walls, sturdy carpeting on the floors, and ceilings made of pressed plastic. But Margaret's furnishings overcame the sterility of the basic decor. Handmade quilts, afghans, pillows, scarves, and doilies adorned the furniture, old but polished and clean. The small, convenient kitchen and bath had bright new appliances, easy to use and to clean, and such safety features as a grab bar on the wall next to the commode and a sit-down shelf on the molded shower wall. Doorways were wide enough to accommodate a wheelchair, should it be needed.

Margaret exuded pride and contentment. "I haven't ever had such new things, not anywhere I've lived. It's a dear little house, and I love taking care of it. And think how nice it is to have Bridget and Bob next door, and the children to drop in on their old granny when they're at home."

Both Bridget and Margaret spoke with admiration about how quickly the cottage had been set in place. "The truck brought it in one morning, and some workmen set it up on the foundation they'd put in a couple of weeks before. Then there was a lot of coming and going by electricians, plumbers, inspectors, who knows what all. By the next evening it was all hooked up and ready for Ma to move in. Incredible!" Gazing out the window at an old apple tree in first bloom, the older woman murmured, "It's lovely. Just lovely."

A prime supporter of ECHO housing, the American Association of Retired Persons (AARP) has mounted a campaign to educate the public about its economic and other benefits. AARP believes the concept can gain community acceptance by emphasizing that "neighborhoods will maintain their character and preserve their quality if local ECHO units are designed to: provide a temporary residence for relatives of the property owner; be removed from the site when they are no longer needed by the relatives of the owner; and compliment the exterior of the original home."

Accessory Apartments and Home Sharing

In chapter 3, I described accessory apartments and home sharing which provided financial and social supports, enabling the home-owner to remain living in the home. These are also options for the older person who wants to move into a rental or become a home sharee.

We met Dorothy in chapter 3, who had converted the second floor of her house into a three-room apartment. She was introduced to Jenny, who at age seventy-six was looking for a place to live, at a county housing agency. Jenny's husband, a barber, had died of a debilitating nerve disease. A gentle and patient woman, she had lovingly nursed him through the last four years of his life while their savings were drained by medical bills. For that reason she was grateful to her only daughter and son-in-law for putting the couple up, rent-free, in a three-room apartment in their two-story home. Soon after the death of Jenny's husband, however, a change of job made it necessary for her son-in-law to sell the house and move his family to a distant part of the state. The couple asked Jenny to move with them but she wanted to stay in the area where she had spent most of her life.

So Jenny's next move was into a room in her son's apartment in the next town. It was small and crowded. "I didn't mind that so much. I had a place for myself for most of the day. But Mike and Sulee hadn't been married very long, and I felt they needed their privacy," Jenny explained, adding that she had lived in many apartments, some large and some quite small, during her married life.

Then a good friend living in the city lost her husband and asked Jenny to come and stay with her for a while. It was only a three-room apartment, so Jenny slept on the couch in the living room. "It was really quite comfortable. And we talked and cried together, remembering old times. I stayed almost a year, until my friend was ready to move south to a retirement place near her daughter's family," Jenny said.

By that time, Mike had found his mother an inexpensive, one-bedroom garden apartment in town. Though not specifically designed for older people, many of the building's tenants were elderly, and they had formed a good, informal social system—looking out for and helping each other. Jenny was happy there, but after only two years the landlord opted for condominium conversion, forcing many of the older tenants to move out.

"That was a blow. For the first time in a long time, I'd allowed myself to feel a sense of permanence," Jenny recalled sadly. "But," she added, "it's all turned out for the best. Because Dorothy was able to convert the upstairs of her house, I have this lovely, roomy apartment. I'm still near my son and Sulee and the children. And I see some of my old friends at the senior center, which I can walk to every day as long as I keep my health. I'm quite content. I just hope I can live here for the rest of my life."

In chapter 3, we also met Martha, who wanted someone to share her home because she was lonely and depressed and needed some homemaking services. Charlotte, a bustling, competent woman of seventy, found she could be useful and earn a little money, too, when she agreed to move into Martha's house.

Charlotte and her husband, who had died a short time before, had been government clerks in Washington, D.C. After his death, she sold their house and moved to Ohio to live with her only daughter, Eve, whose husband was an auto mechanic. There were five grandchildren, all nearly grown, and there was much coming and going in the household. Problems arose when Charlotte tried to impose some order on the chaos, thus antagonizing her son-in-law. Enlisting the help of her daughter, she consulted a housemate-matching service.

Charlotte had very little money to spend on housing. But Martha did not need the money; she was offering two rooms—sitting room and bedroom with bath—plus the run of the living area rent-free. In addition, she would pay $100 per month in exchange for services. What Martha hoped for was an efficient house manager to cook, shop, and organize the household. And that's what she found in Charlotte.

Charlotte was very happy with this living arrangement. She enjoyed being useful to another person and running a household again. She received free room and board and an additional sum every month, all of which was a welcome supplement to her small government pension, enabling her to establish gift funds for her grandchildren, help her daughter with some of the family's financial problems, and buy a few extras for herself. "I am real pleased with the way things worked out," she concluded.

The people I have been describing in this chapter all chose to, or were forced to, move from their homes and find alternative housing. In many of these cases, their situations were no different from those of the other elderly whom we met in the previous chapters who chose to remain living in their own homes. It is obvious that the choices that are made in one's living arrangements as one gets older are determined by many different factors. I will be exploring this topic in the next chapter.

Checking It Out

Guidelines for Making Housing Decisions

I have been exploring different ways and means of continuing to live in one's own home. The previous chapters have dealt with home equity conversion, home sharing, accessory apartments, home maintenance and home repair programs, home safety and security, community services and programs, and information and referral. I have also included a chapter on relocating one's home to a warmer climate.

How do you decide which of these choices are the right ones for you? Obviously, there are no perfect solutions—each person has to carefully weigh the pros and cons of each possibility. And depending on the kind of person you are, your marital status, your income and assets, your health and functional ability, your preferred life-style, and the location of your family and friends, you can plan your housing and living arrangements to suit your individual needs.

Answering the following questions should help in your decision making about whether you ought to remain in your present home and, if you do, what changes you need to make to make your home a better place to live in now and in the future.[1]

A. Home and Neighborhood	Yes	No
1. Do I like my home?		
2. Is it comfortable and pleasant?		

3. Is it the right size?

4. Is it in good repair, both inside and outside?

5. Is the heating system and insulation adequate?

6. Is the neighborhood safe and attractive?

7. Is there good crime control?

8. Is it convenient to stores, banks, etc.?

9. Is it convenient to health and community services and facilities?

10. Can I get to my church or synagogue?

11. Can I get to recreational, cultural, and educational facilities?

12. Am I near family and friends?

13. Do I have someone close by to count on for help in case of emergency?

14. Am I near volunteer and employment opportunities?

15. Are there opportunities for making new friends when old friends move away or die?

16. Are there opportunities for new hobby and recreational pursuits?

17. Does my present location allow me to get enough exercise?

18. Do I like the climate?

19. Is the climate good for my health?

20. Is it important for me to remain in the area?

B. Physical and Financial (Present and Future)   **Yes   No**

1. Is my home safe and hazard-free?

2. Does the physical layout match my functional ability? (e.g., Can I manage stairs? Reach cabinets and shelves?)

3. Is my home easy to maintain? Can I take care of it now?

4. Will I be able to take care of it for the next five to ten years?

5. Does my home (including taxes and utilities) cost more than 30 percent of my income?

6. Will I be able to afford my home over the next five to ten years?

7. Will my home continue to be suitable even if my health or mobility deteriorates?

8. Do I own and drive a car?

9. Can I continue driving over the next five to ten years?

10. Is there public transportation nearby?

C. Personal Feelings   Yes   No

1. Do I feel content and not lonely or isolated in my home?

2. Do I have pleasant feelings and memories associated with my present home?

3. Do I find it difficult to make changes?

4. Do I prefer the familiar rather than new experiences?

5. Is it difficult for me to adjust to new friends and new social situations?

6. Is it difficult for me to meet new challenges?

7. Is privacy very important to me?

8. Is being independent very important to me?

9. Would I feel uncomfortable living in an age-segregated environment?

10. Do I feel that moving would be too stressful?

11. Do I feel that living in retirement housing would make me feel old and more dependent?

12. Would I resent living in a situation in which I would have to obey rules and regulations?

If your answers to most of the above questions are "yes," then you are satisfied with your present housing and obviously wish to continue living in your own home. However, you should probably investigate programs and services that would enrich your life or make it easier, such as a nutrition site, senior center, or volunteer program. This is particularly important for those who said "no" to questions A–12 (Near family and friends?) and C–1 (Content and not lonely?) (see chapters 6 and 7).

If you answered "yes" to most of the questions but "no" to A–4, A–5, B–1, B–2, B–3, B–4, and B–7, you should consider checking out repair services, weatherization, and chore services available to seniors in your community, and measures to improve the safety and security of your home (see chapters 4 and 5).

The person who answered "yes" to most of the questions but "no" to questions B–1, B–2, B–5, B–6, and C–3 should consider some form of home equity conversion (see chapter 2). Receipt of additional income will relieve your high housing cost and provide funds for proper maintenance and repair. Perhaps by means of a reverse mortgage or deferred loan, you can remain in your own home and still solve some of the problems with your house.

Answering "yes" to most of the questions but "no" to A–3, A–12, A–13, A–15, B–5, B–6, B–7, C–1, and C–3 would indicate that you feel lonely and far from family and friends, in a house that is too large, and that you have doubts about being able to maintain and pay for it in the coming years. Add the admission of aversion to change, and you have a combination that calls for consideration of a home-sharing arrangement. Depending on your exact circumstances, you should evaluate home sharing or creating an accessory apartment (see chapter 3). If your answer to question C–7 was "yes," an accessory apartment might be preferable to a sharing arrangement.

If you think adding an accessory apartment or entering into a shared-housing arrangement would be a suitable arrangement for you, then I would suggest that you review the questions in chapter 3. I have introduced these questionnaires not to discourage anyone from pursuing any of these courses of action but rather to make them stop and think about some of the consequences of their decisions. It would be useful at this point to briefly review the pros and cons of some of these housing options.

I will compare home equity conversion, adding an accessory apartment, and home sharing. It is obvious that all three options offer extra income and are helpful financially. However, in the case of home equity conversion, the homeowner loses equity in his or her home so that after a period of time this asset could be greatly reduced in value. Moreover, some areas of the United States do not offer this alternative. In addition, home equity conversion does not supply additional security, companionship, or socialization opportunities unless some of the extra income derived from the process is used for these ends.

Home equity conversion usually involves a long-term contract that is not revocable. It also is not available to renters. RMs are expensive because the interest owed is compounded and accrues quickly so that the equity in the house diminishes rapidly. Therefore, if the homeowner is planning to move at a later date and will need some of the equity to cover the purchase or rental costs of new housing, it would be wise to take a smaller monthly RM payment and conserve some of the equity.

However, home equity conversion does have its positive aspects. The homeowner receives additional income without losing any of his or her privacy or making any changes in the home, and except in the case of a sale leaseback, retains ownership of the home.

In some home equity conversions, particularly for short-term reverse mortgages, the homeowner has to pay off the loan or sell the house. Therefore, if he or she had not planned to move, he or she may be forced to do so in order to pay back the loan. On the other hand, if he or she wants to continue to live in the home for a limited time, this type of loan can enable the homeowner to do so.

The extra income derived from home equity conversion enables the homeowner to make necessary repairs to the house or to purchase housekeeping or home-health services. Another advantage links home equity conversion with the other two choices, since the income produced by home equity conversion can provide the homeowner with the money he or she needs to make any changes to the house. This money could be used to make modifications needed for home sharing or to pay for work needed to create an accessory apartment.

In addition to bringing in extra income, both home sharing and an accessory apartment offer added security by bringing another person in the house to call on in case of emergency. The former option offers opportunities for adding increased socialization, companionship, and services, while the latter option may or may not provide such opportunities.

Home sharing usually involves no changes or very limited changes to the house, while adding an accessory apartment obviously requires extensive renovations. In addition, the latter option reduces the homeowner's living space to a much greater extent than the former option. On the other hand, home sharing requires giving up some of one's privacy in exchange for the advantages mentioned in the previous paragraph. In the case of accessory apartments, the homeowner can choose to live quite separately from his or her tenant, as was illustrated in chapter 3.

A major disadvantage of home sharing, in addition to the loss of privacy, is the problem of finding a compatible housemate. This is becoming less of a problem due to the proliferation of nonprofit public and private house-matching agencies (see chapter 3).

Zoning problems may arise in a home-sharing arrangement, but they are far more likely to occur when adding an accessory apartment—unless the house is located in a two-family zone or the municipality is willing to make exceptions to accommodate the special needs of its elderly residents. Another disadvantage of an accessory apartment is the fact that the homeowner has to find a contractor to make the necessary alterations at a reasonable price. In addition, he or she must live with noise, mess, and other inconveniences during the renovation, and be willing to live thereafter in a reduced space.

It is obvious that both accessory apartments and home sharing do not change the homeowner's status: he or she still retains ownership of the house.

Home equity conversion and adding an accessory apartment are options available only to homeowners. However, if a renter has at least a two-bedroom apartment he or she can consider a home-sharing arrangement.

Of the three options, home sharing can offer the best solution for reducing social isolation and loneliness.

Although I devoted a chapter to the topic of relocating one's home to a warmer climate, I would now like to briefly review some of the pros and cons of such a move. If the home is presently located in a cold climate and the owner has a serious health problem that would be helped by living in the South or the Southwest, then a move to a different area should be seriously considered. Living in the southern part of the country protects the elderly from many of the health hazards posed by the northern climate: cold, raw weather that causes respiratory problems, the dangers of falls caused by ice and snow, colds and flu, etc. Moreover, the milder southern climate allows people to be outdoors almost every day, all year round. Homes cost less in the South and the Southwest, and maintenance expenses and taxes are lower than in the North. The southern and southwestern life-styles are less hectic than in the North.

Although some of the relocatees found an added advantage of being closer to children or other family members when they moved south, most were actually living further away from their family. Although they continued to stay in contact by returning north on a regular basis and by having their children occasionally visit them, many of the elderly found distance from family and infrequent family contact to be a major deterrent to relocating.

Another disadvantage to changing one's place of residence is the emotional and physical stress and strain involved in selling one's house, sorting all one's possessions and furnishings, packing, finding a new place to live, and refurnishing. For many elderly these stresses can outweigh the advantages of a move to a warmer climate.

Before a decision is made to relocate, you need to spend some time—at least a month—trying out the new area. It is best that you spend several different periods of time over the course of the year to make sure that both the climate and the housing in the new area are acceptable to you.

Before I end this chapter, let us return to Susan, an elderly widow whom we first met in chapter 1, and guess what her responses would be to the initial set of questions posed at the beginning of this chapter. You may recall that Susan lives alone in a seven-room ranch house and is an active and extremely intelligent woman who is in relatively good health and still drives her own car. She is involved in community work and continues to serve on several important local government councils.

Since she loved her home of so many years and found it convenient to family and friends and to her hobby interests and volunteer activities, she would probably have answered "yes" to most, if not all, of the questions listed under "A. Home and Neighborhood." Reviewing the next set of questions under "B. Physical and Financial: Present and Future," she would probably have answered "yes" to 1, 2, 3, 6, and 8, and "no" to 4, 5, 7, 9, and 10. In "C. Personal Feelings," her responses to 1, 2, 3, 4, 7, 8, 9, 10, 11, and 12 would probably be "yes," and "no" to 5 and 6.

If Susan were to plan for the future, she could take comfort from her financial situation. She faces no financial problems in continuing to remain in her own home. Therefore, since she has sufficient income, she would not need any type of home equity conversion, or the financial assistance of a weatherization, life-line, or other community maintenance or repair services.

However, since she is now finding the outside work and gardening more difficult, she might want to explore a chore service in her town. Her degree of frailty might worsen in the coming years so that she should consider installing some safety measures in her home, such as grab bars in the bathrooms. She probably would not consider having a housemate because of her need for privacy but could consider creating an accessory apartment since there are seven rooms and an unfinished basement in her house.

If she rejects this last option, she could probably benefit from telephone reassurance and friendly visitor programs in the future.

Now that I have explored the major housing choices presently available to the elderly who prefer to remain living in their own homes, I want to end the book by discussing what the future may hold.

A Look to the Future

New Pilot Programs, Such as Life-Care-At-Home, and Proposed Federal Housing Legislation

Based on the projected older population in the next few decades, we can assume that there will be a marked increase in the numbers of those sixty-five and older and an even greater increase of those over seventy-five. The elderly will be better educated and more sophisticated, and probably will be better off financially, than the present elderly. In addition, their children will more likely be living further away from them. As more and more women take jobs outside the home, fewer homemaker daughters will be available as caregivers for their aging parents. But with increased longevity, the elderly will become more frail and more prone to serious illnesses requiring more care as they become very old.

In light of the present trend of older people wanting to live independently and separately from their adult children, we can anticipate that they will need more community supports and greater changes in their housing design, including more safety and security measures for the home. The growing number of people of advanced old age with limited functional capacities may force them to move in with adult children or enter nursing homes prematurely (neither decision as a first choice), unless they have planned for some acceptable alternatives at an earlier time.

Tools and Devices

There is now a growing awareness on the part of both the aging agencies and the community at large that it is important to help older people make their homes safer and more secure. As I discussed in chapter 5, the New Jersey Home Security and Transportation program, which provides for greater security by offering double locks for front and back doors, etc., at no cost or only a nominal cost, has become a model for the rest of the country. This very simple and inexpensive service has proved to be very important to the people it has served and will probably become available in most areas.

Many companies are developing simple devices for people who live alone and want to be able to summon help in case of emergencies. One simple device is called Life Alert. It consists of a vial that can be attached to the refrigerator or the dashboard of the car. The vial contains a person's important medical information—doctors' names and telephone numbers, blood type, allergies, prescribed medications, special health needs, etc.—and can be very useful in a health emergency. These vials are very inexpensive and their universal distribution would save many lives each year. Area agencies on aging usually buy and distribute Life Alert vials to the elderly populations they serve.

Also, there has been an increase in the manufacturing of tools and devices to help handicapped and older persons manage by themselves in their own homes. Whirlpool, as one example, has produced a booklet on techniques for reaching and handling stoves, ovens, sinks, and other kinds of food preparation devices (see chapter 5). A motorized kitchen has been designed in Sweden and is available through an office in Saskatchewan, Canada. It has countertops and kitchen appliances driven by electric motors.[1]

An interesting bathtub-shower unit is distributed by Bathease Inc. of Tampa, Florida. It is made of fiberglass and has a watertight door so that the older person can step into the unit without having to step over a shower sill or the side of a bathtub. The barrier-free entrance is much safer than the standard tub or shower. The unit is designed so that grab bars can be easily installed.[2]

"Touch-on" devices make turning lights on and off easier because they require less hand movement. Available for new or old lamps, the devices are sold by Sears, Roebuck, other catalogue stores, and local department stores.[3]

Royal Doulton, a British manufacturer of fine china, has introduced cups, saucers, glasses, and flatware that require less strength and less motor coordination on the part of the users. They are so subtly designed that the differences between these new dishware, glasses, and utensils and the ordinary ones are not very obvious.[4]

Many other innovative tools and devices to aid the elderly consumer are coming on the market all the time. Meanwhile, architects and gerontologists using our rapidly expanding technology are beginning to explore "Smart Houses" for older people.[5] The idea is to give the elderly better control over their immediate environment. Through advances in electronics, computers, and robots it is anticipated that a person could turn appliances on and off by verbal command. Homes could be redesigned to compensate for losses in vision, hearing, touch, smell, memory, and mobility. Smart Houses would not only improve older people's independence but would also add to their quality of life; using less of their energy for household chores, they would have more energy for social and recreational activities.

Federal legislation has been introduced that provides for a two-year grant program to local governments and nonprofit organizations to provide home repairs to low-income elderly. "Eligible repairs include preventive repairs, security-related measures, accessibility and suitability repairs, and general repairs."[6]

I anticipate that home sharing will become much more common as homematch agencies proliferate and become more skillful and experienced in making matches. I have already noted the present dramatic increase in this type of living arrangement (see chapter 3). This housing alternative should be more acceptable to the next generation of older people who have had more experience with shared living. Also, more of the elderly will be forced to consider this kind of living arrangement as they advance in age and lose "hands-on" family support due to their children's dispersion across America.

Upgrading Neighborhoods

Dr. Robert W. Taylor describes a very interesting pilot program in Clifton, New Jersey, that addresses the financial needs of the low- and moderate-income elderly living in old neighborhoods.[7] Because escalating rents have produced a hardship for the older renters, a partnership has been developed among the renters, the landlords, and the city that has produced significantly lower rents for the seniors. This arrangement is based on the proposition that seniors are a stabilizing force in the community and should be helped to continue to live in the area. Since many of the landlords are long-time owners of their properties and their mortgages are paid off, they can more easily afford to lower rents; some actually gain by the resultant reduced turnover. The city is using federal Community Development funds to improve these neighborhoods by putting in new sidewalks, curbs, streetlights, and other forms of improvements which include added crime prevention programs. The program provides the elderly with immediate, direct savings in the form of rent reductions, indirectly helps the landlord since it increases the value of his property over the long term, and makes the community a better place to live in for all its residents.

Although I am not aware of any replication of this program in any other state, it should not be too difficult to develop in other areas where large numbers of low- to moderate-income elderly renters exist and some type of federal or state funding is available.

Fannie Mae Low-Cost Mortgages

A new program was announced in 1989 by Fannie Mae, a private company chartered by Congress to provide low-cost mortgages to people of low, moderate, or middle incomes. This new demonstration project will test several housing alternatives for the elderly, including accessory apartments and home sharing.[8]

An accessory apartment is one alternative for the homeowner who lives alone, needs extra income, and wants to have another person living in the house in case of an emergency (see chapter 3). Fannie Mae is offering a mortgage to any person who is sixty-two years of age or older. In the case of a couple, at least one spouse must qualify. The homeowner can borrow enough cash out of the equity in his house to finance the accessory apartment renovation. Some of the rental income can then be used to repay the loan.

If older homeowners want to share their homes and need refinancing to make necessary changes, Fannie Mae will allow the income to be received from the home sharees in calculating the applicant's eligibility for a mortgage. Fannie Mae will consider any type of home sharing, but prefers one that involves a home-match agency. Fannie Mae will also finance sale leasebacks (see chapter 2), for up to 90 percent of the value of the house. Anyone interested in participating in this program must contact one of the regional Fannie Mae offices.[9]

Insured RMs

In spite of the Fannie Mae program in regard to sale leasebacks, the present trend in home equity conversions would seem to be to reverse mortgages (RM) (see chapter 2). The introduction of federally insured RMs has given this program a real boost; it is presently available in almost forty states. Because of the initial interest in the insured RMs, new legislation has been introduced increasing the number from the present 2,500 limit to 25,000. This federal program not only offers several types of RMs but also the most flexibility since the older person is not locked into just one option but can change or combine different kinds of RMs.

Although the elderly have been reluctant to use home equity conversions as a means of acquiring additional income, new federal programs could encourage more elderly to use this option. AARP is analyzing all the available RMs in the United States and expects to publish a report by the end of 1990.

Mark R. Meiners in a chapter in *Aging in Place* has suggested that with the increased need for home-based services HECs might be combined with long-term-care insurance to help pay for home care. He feels that this option might be particularly appealing to the low- and moderate-income elderly who at the present time cannot afford the cost of long-term-care insurance.[10]

Support Services

Since it is projected that the elderly population is growing at an accelerating pace and that this is particularly true for the older-old, it is obvious that there will be an increasing need for support services in order to enable them to remain at home. Two solutions have been suggested, but neither has yet been put into practice. One suggestion is that the senior citizen subsidized housing projects that offer support services should open up these services to other older people who live in the neighborhood. If the project provides meals and/or recreational programs, for example, nearby residents could be transported by means of shuttle buses to the project. Housekeeping and other support services could be offered on a fee-for-service basis or as a complete package. Not only would this help some of the area elderly remain in their own homes, but it should increase community acceptance of the subsidized housing projects.[11]

A second idea to help people continue to live in their own homes has been proposed by the author. This concept is based on congregate housing service subsidies that are funded by the federal government and some of the states. This program provides service subsidies to tenants living in senior housing projects who need meals, housekeeping, and some assistance with daily living in order to remain independent. It has proven to be extremely successful. In New Jersey, for example, this program started about 11 years ago with approximately two hundred people and is now serving well over twelve hundred. It has helped many people who wanted to remain in the housing project by delaying or totally eliminating the need to move in with children or enter a nursing home.

Many apartment buildings and garden complexes contain a significant number of elderly tenants who have aged in place. I do not know how many of these people are in need of similar services available to elders living in subsidized housing or how many could pay for them. However, in many communities these services are not readily available or the older persons in need are not able to get to them. It should be possible for a family service or other community agency, with some financial support as a start-up, to rent one of the apartments in a subsidized project building to use as a communal dining room and drop-in center for the tenants who have paid for these congregate services. Although, as I indicated earlier, such services are not yet available to renters in a nonsubsidized, private rental complex, I feel that this will be a new trend in the delivery of support services.

Recently, the Robert Wood Johnson Foundation has initiated a demonstration program in 11 states to integrate the delivery of nonmedical services by home-health agencies.[12] It is called the Supportive Services Program for Older Persons (SSPOP). The funding will run through 1991, after which time it is expected that the programs will be self-supporting since the clients pay for the services received. The SSPOP provides for the delivery of house-based services such as minor home repairs, chore services, home maintenance, lawn and yard maintenance, housekeeping and housecleaning, and transportation where they previously did not exist. It also offers case management and caregiver education and counseling. The uniqueness of this program is that a single agency, a home-health-care agency, is coordinating its traditional health services with all the other house-related services needed by the elderly persons they serve.

In its first year of operation, the SSPOP has serviced about 3,000 people at the 11 sites. It has provided the frail and home-bound elderly with more control over their physical environment and enabled them to remain living in their own homes.

Life-Care-at-Home

The most promising new trend in housing options to help people stay in their own homes is being tested in four places in the country: Philadelphia; Delaware County, Pennsylvania; Pasadena, California; and Newport News, Virginia. It is called Life-Care-at-Home (LCAH) and guarantees a full range of health and support services for the life of the individual, similar to a Life-Care/Continuing Care Retirement Community. This program not only offers a continuum of services to older people who do not want to move to an LCC/CCRC but it supplies these services at a substantially lower cost. This pilot project is also being funded by the Robert Wood Johnson Foundation.[13]

To help my readers better understand the LCAH, I will describe the model being developed in the northeastern part of Philadelphia by the Jeanes/Foulkeways Corporation, a joint venture between a CCRC and a health-care system that consists of a hospital, nursing home, and home-care agency. The Philadelphia LCAH will provide for a full continuum of services under a life contract.[14] In general, the guaranteed services that are covered under this contract are acute care and physician care, one hundred days of short-term personal and skilled nursing care, one hundred days of long-term personal and skilled nursing care (patient pays 30 percent of any additional care in a semiprivate room), home health care, home health assistance/homemaker service, emergency response system, social and medical day care ($5 per day copayment), home-delivered meals ($1 per meal copayment), biannual home inspection, and many social/recreational activities. Some are included in the monthly fee while others involve a copayment.

Other benefits are offered on a fee-for-service basis and are not included in the monthly charge. These include home maintenance, lawn service, snow removal, a travel club, and financial and legal planning.

Only those people who are in relatively good health and living independently are eligible for admission to this plan. Similar to an LCC/CCRC, an LCAH includes both an entry fee and a monthly charge. Upon the death of a member in the plan, no refund of either of these fees is returned to the heir(s). However, if a member chooses to withdraw from the plan, a portion of the entry fee will be refunded (for each month the person has been in the plan 2 percent of the entry fee will be deducted. After fifty months the entry fee becomes nonrefundable).

The entry fee has two categories, one for people aged 65–74, and the other for those aged 75–85. Initially, the plan will not admit anyone over the age of 85. A couple pays about 10 percent less than two individuals paying separately. Two optional payment plans are projected. One will have a higher entry fee and lower monthly payments, while the other will be just the reverse.

At the time of this writing, about 116 older people are enrolled in the plan, with many more "waiting in the wings" to see it in operation first. Jeanes/Foulkeways had hoped to have two hundred in the plan before they began but are now considering starting the program with the present number of enrollees.

Now I would like to introduce some of the people who have enrolled in LCAH.[15] Bob and Lois O'Dell are a couple who met fifty-five years ago in high school. Bob went on to college and became a chemist, while his wife obtained a degree in education. She is presently employed as financial secretary of a foundation; Bob retired 11 years ago from a pharmaceutical company. They are both active in their church. Lois O'Dell serves on the board of directors of a number of social service children's agencies and is also the corresponding secretary of her high school alumni association and editor of its newsletter. Her husband's hobbies include bicycling, astronomy, electronics, and computers. They have been married almost forty-eight years and have two married sons and four grandsons. Mr. and Mrs. O'Dell want to remain living in their own home and feel that the LCAH plan with its homemaking, house maintenance, and health services will allow them to do this for many years to come.

Another couple, Leonard and Elinor Winston, were also attracted to the plan because they felt that it would enable them to remain at home and continue their active life-style. Leonard is a former trustee of a college and presently serves as a trustee of his local congregation, is a member of his township's citizen board, and of the senior activities center board. He is a college graduate and a former executive. He is an avid golfer and enjoys taking courses at several local colleges. Elinor has a degree in psychology and has worked as a librarian and been a volunteer tutor. She is very interested in current events and enjoys reading and needlepoint. Both she and her husband share an interest in early American furnishings and are members of the National Trust for Historic Preservation.

Dr. and Mrs. Clark are a very interesting older couple who are avid gardeners and world travelers. They have accumulated many unusual collectibles from their trips. He is a retired hospital psychiatrist and she is a former high school counselor. They are both Quakers and the fact that the LCAH plan is administered by a Quaker organization was an important factor in their choice of this plan. However, the more important consideration was that although they have three children and eight grandchildren, their family lives too far away to provide any support services. They both think that they will need some additional help if they want to remain at home. Dr. Clark feels that the LCAH will "assure us of good medical care as long as we live."

Some single older people have become charter members of the plan. Elizabeth Miller has lived in her present house for forty years and wants to continue to live there as long as possible. She retired in 1984 after a long career as a religious educator. Her last position was as director of education for a group of parishes. She was raised in Utah, the daughter of a missionary among the Indians. Her husband died almost three years ago, and she decided to become involved in her church in a new way. She organized a committee on older adults within her parish and has remained actively involved in it. She is also very fond of music and plays the recorder in a quartet and teaches the recorder to students. Like so many of the people we have met in this book, Elizabeth and her husband built the house she now lives in and it represents many important memories and family experiences to her.

Eldercare

Another interesting service in helping the elderly remain in their homes is provided by employers who recognize that many of their employees are caregivers for their parents and need help in maintaining their dual roles. Currently only a small number of companies are providing some form of "eldercare" assistance to their workers, but this benefit will become more popular as more employers become aware of their employees' reduced effectiveness due to the stress of caregiving.

The types of eldercare services provided range from dissemination of information, to referral and counseling service, to arranging on-site day care for elderly parents, to offering liberal leave policies and flexible work options.[16]

Community Resources

Now that I have outlined some of the newer and more experimental housing programs that can enable older people to remain in their own homes, let me recapitulate the various community resources that were mentioned throughout the book, particularly in chapters 6 and 7. As I indicated, the state and area agencies on aging should be your starting point for information, referral, and any other kind of housing assistance you may need. In addition, family counseling and service agencies, mental health agencies, senior centers, geriatric care managers, and housing agencies can often help in solving housing problems. Religious and ethnic organizations may also be useful resources. (See appendices for addresses and telephone numbers of agencies and organizations.)

A new consumer-oriented program has been developed by the AARP in cooperation with the Administration on Aging. It is called Consumer Housing Information Service for Seniors (CHISS). It began as a pilot program in a few places a couple of years ago but has now become a full-fledged program in twenty-five states. Its goal is to become operative throughout the country by the end of 1990.

The AARP is administering the CHISS program. It works through a lead agency in each locality, usually the state or area agency on aging. With this agency's cooperation, the AARP trains volunteers in housing programs, resources, and other related information.

These CHISS volunteers are called Housing Information Volunteers (HIVs) and they provide information to older people or their families about all the various housing programs and options that exist in their communities.[17]

The HIVs are available on a one-to-one basis, can come to the person's home for one or more consultations, and offer their services free of charge. These volunteers do not give advice or counseling on a housing problem; they merely offer information, answer questions, and clarify misunderstandings about the various housing programs and options open to the individual homeowner or apartment dweller. Where necessary, they will refer the senior to an appropriate source for counseling or more specific help. If you do not know if or where a CHISS exists in your area, you should contact your local area agency on aging or the AARP in Washington, D.C.

As you have seen, many programs and resources exist to assist older people to remain in their own homes. However, not every kind of program is offered in every area, several are income-restricted or limited to special categories of applicants, and others may have long waiting lists. In addition, some programs described in this book may not be available in the future due to budgetary cutbacks at the federal and state levels.

If now or in the future you could be interested in a specific housing program or service I have discussed and it is not available in your area, you and/or your family might try to stimulate the local governing body to explore appropriate housing alternatives and supports in order to keep the elderly in the community. Get senior center participants, older members of your congregation, and members of local service clubs to apply additional pressure on the government. Try to influence your church, synagogue, or local service club to initiate a house-match program, a home maintenance service, a chore service, or some other program that will aid the elderly in your community.

Mary and Her Aunt Margaret

Before I end this book I should like to share a story with you that my friend Mary told me about her Aunt Margaret. This aunt is eighty-one years old and lives in a two-bedroom, two-bath condominium. She was widowed twice; her first marriage lasted twenty-four years and her second twenty years. Her second husband died eleven years ago. Both her children, a married daughter and a bachelor son, live in the North.

Aunt Margaret's first husband was an attorney and her second a retired businessman. She, herself, was an elementary schoolteacher. According to Mary, her aunt is an unusually attractive woman with an easy-going, pleasant personality. She drives a car and plays golf several times a week. In addition to the golf, she takes a brisk forty-minute walk each morning and attends exercise class four times a week. She is an avid card player and plays bridge and canasta with her women friends very frequently. She also has many cultural interests, and attends the theater, concerts, and dance programs.

About a year ago, Aunt Margaret had a small stroke. She seemed to recover physically, but it left her with some memory loss. Her driving is somewhat impaired and she is nervous and does not handle traffic very well. She insists on driving in spite of these difficulties because it is very important for her to be independent.

My friend Mary is very fond of Margaret and visits her each winter. She told me that on her recent visit she was very troubled by the changes she observed in her aunt's behavior. "Although she has always been a very gracious hostess, this time her kitchen seemed quite disorganized. There was very little food in the house. She buys only a few items at a time or forgets to shop altogether. I am not sure whether she is eating properly or regularly and I am quite concerned about her," Mary said.

Margaret has become aware of her memory loss and finds the problem most disturbing. She has always prided herself on her excellent health and physical condition and seems quite depressed about her present level of functioning. She wants to continue living in her own home. She will not consider moving in with either of her children although either would be pleased to have her.

Mary confided to me: "The last time she was up North, she seemed disoriented away from home and became easily flustered. She forgot dates and became confused about specific times and days. But the behavior that worries me the most is that I have begun to notice some changes in her personality that are alarming. She has always been an extremely kind and considerate person but now she is very short-tempered, nervous, depressed, and can be quite disagreeable."

On Mary's last visit, she tried to interest her aunt in making some changes in her present living arrangement, such as having a housemate or moving to a more supportive environment such as a congregate or life-care facility. She said, "One minute, Aunt Margaret was very receptive and would agree to explore these possibilities and the next time she would change completely and say, 'I'm not ready for that.'"

Mary feels that her aunt cannot cope with her present situation nor plan for her future in a rational manner. "If she doesn't make some changes in her housing fairly soon, she will continue to deteriorate and may not have any choice left except a nursing home." However, Mary felt that it was highly unlikely that her aunt would be able to make any suitable decision.

Mary's Aunt Margaret is a good example of an older woman who was still in good health in her late seventies but who failed to plan for any changes in her housing arrangements to accommodate any frailties or functional limitations in her later years. A few years ago, Margaret would have been able to explore many different living arrangements. At that time she might very well have decided to share her house with someone who would initially just be a housemate but later on could have helped her with the driving, shopping, and cooking. With such an arrangement, Margaret might be able to live out the rest of life in her own home.

Since none of us can be sure of what our future holds in terms of loss of family and friends, degree of frailty, and health, it becomes even more important to examine all our housing and living arrangement options while we still have the energy and ability to do so. Planning for our later years at the appropriate time allows us to continue to have control over our lives and to continue to live independently.

Appendix I: State Units on Aging

ALABAMA
Commission on Aging
136 Catoma Street
Montgomery, AL 36130
205/242–5743

ALASKA
Older Alaskans Commission
Department of Administration
Pouch C-Mail Station 0209
Juneau, AK 99811–0209
907/465–3250

ARIZONA
Aging and Adult
   Administration
Department of Economic
   Security
1400 West Washington Street
Phoenix, AZ 85007
602/542–4446

ARKANSAS
Division of Aging & Adult
   Services
Arkansas Department of
   Human Services
P. O. Box 1417, SLOT 1412
7th and Main Streets
Little Rock, AR 72201
501/682–2441

CALIFORNIA
Department of Aging
1600 K Street
Sacramento, CA 95814
916/322–5290

COLORADO
Aging & Adult Services
Department of Social Services
1575 Sherman Street, 10th
   Floor
Denver, CO 80203–1714
303/866–3851

CONNECTICUT
Department on Aging
175 Main Street
Hartford, CT 06106
203/566–3238

DELAWARE
Division on Aging
Department of Health &
   Social Services
1901 North DuPont Highway
New Castle, DE 19720
302/421–6791

DISTRICT OF COLUMBIA
Office on Aging
1424 K Street, N.W.
2nd Floor
Washington, DC 20005
202/724–5626

FLORIDA
Program Office of Aging &
  Adult Services
Department of Health &
  Rehabilitative Services
1317 Winewood Boulevard
Tallahassee, FL 32301
904/488–8922

GEORGIA
Office of Aging
878 Peachtree Street, N.E.
Room 632
Atlanta, GA 30309
404/894–5333

GUAM
Division of Senior Citizens
Department of Public Health
  & Social Services
Government of Guam
Post Office Box 2816
Agana, GU 96910

HAWAII
Executive Office on Aging
Office of the Governor
335 Merchant Street
Room 241
Honolulu, HI 96813
808/548–2593

IDAHO
Office on Aging
Room 114, Statehouse
Boise, ID 83720
208/334–3833

ILLINOIS
Department on Aging
421 East Capitol Avenue
Springfield, IL 62701
217/785–2870

INDIANA
Division of Aging Services
Department of Human
  Services
251 North Illinois Street
P. O. Box 7083
Indianapolis, IN 46207–7083
317/232–7020

IOWA
Department of Elder Affairs
Suite 236, Jewett Building
914 Grand Avenue
Des Moines, IA 50319
515/281–5187

KANSAS
Department on Aging
Docking State Office Building,
  122–S
915 S.W. Harrison
Topeka, KS 66612–1500
913/296–4986

KENTUCKY
Division of Aging Services
Cabinet for Human Resources
CHR Building—6th West
275 East Main Street
Frankfort, KY 40621
502/564–6930

LOUISIANA
Office of Elderly Affairs
4550 N. Boulevard
P. O. Box 80374
Baton Rouge, LA 70806
504/925–1700

MAINE
Bureau of Elder & Adult
  Services
Department of Human
  Services
State House—Station #11
Augusta, ME 04333
207/289–2561

MARYLAND
Office on Aging
State Office Building
301 West Preston Street, Rm.
  1004
Baltimore, MD 21201
301/225–1100

MASSACHUSETTS
Executive Office of
  Elder Affairs
38 Chauncy Street
Boston, MA 02111
617/727–7750

MICHIGAN
Office of Services to the Aging
P.O. Box 30026
Lansing, MI 48909
517/373–8230

MINNESOTA
Board on Aging
Human Services Building
444 Lafayette Road
St. Paul, MN 55255–3843
612/296–2770

MISSISSIPPI
Council on Aging
Division of Aging
  & Adult Services
421 West Pascagoula Street
Jackson, MS 39203
601/354–6100

MISSOURI
Division on Aging
Department of Social Services
P.O. Box 1337—2701 West
  Main St.
Jefferson City, MO 65102
314/751–3082

MONTANA
Department of Family Services
48 North Last Chance Gulch
P.O. Box 8005
Helena, MT 59604
406/444–5900

NEBRASKA
Department on Aging
P.O. Box 95044
301 Centennial Mall-South
Lincoln, NE 68509
402/471–2306

NEVADA
Division for Aging Services
Department of Human
   Resources
340 North 11th Street
Las Vegas, NV 89101
702/486–3545

NEW HAMPSHIRE
Division of Elderly & Adult
   Services
6 Hazen Drive
Concord, NH 03301–6501
603/271–4680

NEW JERSEY
Division on Aging
Department of Community
   Affairs
CN 807
South Broad & Front Streets
Trenton, NJ 08625–0807
609/292–4833

NEW MEXICO
State Agency on Aging
224 East Palace Avenue
La Villa Rivera Building
Santa Fe, NM 87501
505/827–7640

NEW YORK
Office for the Aging
New York State Plaza
Agency Building #2
Albany, NY 12223
518/474–4425

NORTH CAROLINA
Division of Aging
1985 Umstead Dr./Kirby
   Building
Raleigh, NC 27603
919/733–3983

NORTH DAKOTA
Aging Services
Department of Human
   Services
State Capitol Building
Bismarck, ND 58505
701/224–2577

**NORTHERN MARIANA
ISLANDS**
Office of Aging
Department of Community &
   Cultural Affairs
Civic Center—Susupe
Saipan, TT 96950
Tel. Nos. 9411 or 9732

OHIO
Department of Aging
50 West Broad Street
Columbus, OH 43266–0501
614/466–5500

OKLAHOMA
Aging Services Division
Department of Human
  Services
P.O. Box 25352
Oklahoma City, OK 73125
405/521–2281

OREGON
Senior Services Division
313 Public Service Building
Salem, OR 97310
503/378–4728

PENNSYLVANIA
Department of Aging
231 State Street
Harrisburg, PA 17101–1195
717/783–1550

PUERTO RICO
Gericulture Commission
Department of Social Services
Apartado 11398
Santurce, PR 00910
809/721–4010

RHODE ISLAND
Department of Elderly Affairs
160 Pine Street
Providence, RI 02903
401/277–2858

(AMERICAN) SAMOA
Territorial Administration on
  Aging
Office of the Governor
Pago Pago, AS 96799
011 684/633–1252

SOUTH CAROLINA
Commission on Aging
Suite B–500
400 Arbor Lake Drive
Columbia, SC 29223
803/735–0210

SOUTH DAKOTA
Office of Adult Services &
  Aging
700 North Illinois Street
Kneip Building
Pierre, SD 57501
605/773–3656

TENNESSEE
Commission on Aging
Suite 201
706 Church Street
Nashville, TN 37219–5573
615/741–2056

TEXAS
Department on Aging
P.O. Box 12786 Capitol
  Station
1949 IH 35, South
Austin, TX 78741–3702
512/444–2727

**FEDERATED STATES OF
MICRONESIA**
Federated States of Micronesia
Department of Human
  Resources
Kolonia, Pohnpei FM 96941
691/320–2733

UTAH
Division of Aging &
  Adult Services
Department of Social Services
120 North–200 West
Box 45500
Salt Lake City, UT 84145–
  0500
801/538–3910

VERMONT
Department of Rehabilitation
  & Aging
103 South Main Street
Waterbury, VT 05676
802/241–2400

VIRGINIA
Department for the Aging
700 Centre, 10th Floor
700 East Franklin Street
Richmond, VA 23219–2327
804/225–2271

VIRGIN ISLANDS
Senior Citizen Affairs
Department of Human
  Services
#19 Estate Diamond
  Fredericksted
St. Croix, VI 00840
809/772–4950, ext. 46

WASHINGTON
Aging & Adult Services
  Administration
Department of Social &
  Health Services
OB–44A
Olympia, WA 98504
206/586–3768

WEST VIRGINIA
Commission on Aging
Holly Grove—State Capitol
Charleston, WV 25305
304/348–3317

WISCONSIN
Bureau of Aging
Division of Community
  Services
217 South Hamilton Street,
  Suite 300
Madison, WI 53707
608/266–2536

WYOMING
Commission on Aging
Hathaway Building—Room
  139
Cheyenne, WY 82002–0710
307/777–7986

Appendix II: State Housing Finance Agencies

**Alabama Housing Finance
Authority**
P.O. Box 230909
2000 Interstate Park Drive,
   Suite 408
Montgomery, AL 36123–0909
205/242–4310

**Alaska Housing Finance
Corporation**
520 East 34th Street
Anchorage, AK 99503
907/561–1900

**Arizona Department of
Commerce**
Office of Housing
   Development
1700 West Washington, 5th
   Floor
Phoenix, AZ 85007
602/542–5000

**Arkansas Development
Finance Authority**
P.O. Box 8023
100 Main Street, Suite 200
Little Rock, AR 72203
501/682–5900

**California Housing Finance
Agency**
1121 L. Street, 7th Floor
Sacramento, CA 95814
916/322–3991

**Colorado Housing & Finance
Authority**
1981 Blake Street
Denver, CO 80202–1275
303/297–4302

**Connecticut Housing Finance
Authority**
40 Cold Spring Road
Rocky Hill, CT 06067–4005
203/721–9501

**Washington, D.C. Housing
Finance Agency**
1401 New York Avenue, NW,
   Suite 540
Washington, D.C. 20005
202/628–0311

**Delaware State Housing
Authority**
18 The Green
Dover, DE 19901
302/736–4263

Florida Housing Finance Agency
2740 Centerview Drive, Suite 300
Tallahassee, FL 32399–2100
904/488–4197

Georgia Residential Finance Authority
60 Executive Parkway South, Suite 250
Atlanta, GA 30329
404/894–3334

Hawaii Housing Finance & Development Corporation
7 Waterfront Plaza
500 Ala Moana Boulevard, Suite 300
Honolulu, HI 96813
808/543–2987

Idaho Housing Agency
750 W. Myrtle
Boise, ID 83702
208/336–0161

Illinois Housing Finance Authority
401 North Michigan Avenue, Suite 900
Chicago, IL 60611
312/836–5200

Indiana Housing Finance Authority
One N. Capitol Avenue, Suite 515
Indianapolis, IN 46204
317/232–7777

Iowa Finance Authority
200 East Grand Avenue, Suite 222
Des Moines, IA 50309
515/281–4058

Kansas Department of Commerce
400 S.W. Eighth Street
5th Floor
Topeka, KS 66603
913/296–3480

Kentucky Housing Corporation
1231 Louisville Road
Frankfort, KY 40601
502/564–7630

Louisiana Housing Finance Agency
5615 Corporate Boulevard, Suite 6A
Baton Rouge, LA 70808
504/925–3675

Maine State Housing Authority
P.O. Box 2669
295 Water Street
Augusta, ME 04330
207/626–4600

Maryland Community Development Administration
45 Calvert Street
Annapolis, MD 21401
301/974–3161

**Massachusetts Housing
Finance Agency**
50 Milk Street
Boston, MA 02109
617/451–3480

**Michigan State Housing
Development Authority**
401 S. Washington Square
Plaza One Building, 4th Floor
Lansing, MI 48909
517/373–8370

**Minnesota Housing Finance
Agency**
400 Sibley Street, Suite 300
St. Paul, MN 55101
612/296–7608

**Mississippi Home
Corporation**
Dickson Building
510 George Street, Suite 204
Jackson, MS 39201
601/961–4514

**Missouri Housing
Development Commission**
3770 Broadway
Kansas City, MO 64111
816/756–3790

Montana Board of Housing
2001 11th Avenue
Helena, MT 59620
406/444–3040

**Nebraska Investment Finance
Authority**
1033 "O" Street, Suite 218
Lincoln, NE 68508
402/477–4406

Nevada Housing Division
1050 E. William, Suite 435
Carson City, NV 89710
702/885–4258

**New Hampshire Housing
Finance Authority**
24 Constitution Drive
Bedford, NH 03102
603/472–8623

**New Jersey Housing &
Mortgage Finance Agency**
3625 Quakerbridge Road
CN 18550
Trenton, NJ 08650–2085
609/890–8900

**New Mexico Mortgage
Finance Authority**
344 Fourth Street, SW
Albuquerque, NM 87103
505/843–6880

**New York City Housing
Development Corporation**
75 Maiden Lane, 8th Floor
New York, NY 10038
212/344–8080

New York State Division of
Housing & Community
Renewal
38–40 State Street
Albany, NY 12207
212/519–5840

New York State Housing
Finance Agency
Three Park Avenue
New York, NY 10016
212/686–9700

New York State Mortgage
Loan Enforcement & Adm.
Corp.
11 West 42nd Street
New York, NY 10036
212/790–2400

North Carolina Housing
Finance Agency
P.O. Box 28066
Raleigh, NC 27611
919/781–6115

North Dakota Housing
Finance Agency
P.O. Box 1535
1600 E. Interstate Avenue
Bismarck, ND 58501
701/224–3434

Ohio Housing Finance Agency
77 South High Street, 26th
Floor
Columbus, OH 43215
614/466–7970

Oklahoma Housing Finance
Agency
P.O. Box 26720
Oklahoma City, OK 73126–
6720
405/848–1144

Oregon Housing Agency
1600 State Street, Suite 100
Salem, OR 97310–0161
503/378–4343

Pennsylvania Housing Finance
Agency
P.O. Box 8029
2101 North Front Street,
Building #2
Harrisburg, PA 17105–8029
717/780–3800

Puerto Rico Housing Bank &
Finance Agency
P.O. Box 345
606 Barbosa Avenue
Hato Rey, PR 00919
809/765–2537

Puerto Rico Housing Finance
Corp.
Box 42001, Minillas Station
San Juan, PR 00940
809/722–5060

Rhode Island Housing and
Mortgage Finance
Corporation
60 Eddy Street, 2nd Floor
Providence, RI 02903
401/751–5566

**South Carolina State Housing
Finance & Develop. Authority**
1710 Gervais Street, Suite 300
Columbia, SC 29201
803/734–8831

**South Dakota Housing
Development Authority**
P.O. Box 1237
Pierre, SD 57501–1237
605/773–3181

**State of New York Mortgage
Agency**
260 Madison Avenue
New York, NY 10016
212/340–4200

**Tennessee Housing
Development Agency**
700 Landmark Center
401 Church Street
Nashville, TN 37219
615/741–2473

Texas Housing Agency
P.O. Box 13941, Capitol
   Station
Austin, TX 78711–3941
512/474–2974

Utah Housing Finance Agency
177 East 100 South
Salt Lake City, UT 84111
801/521–6950

**Vermont Housing Finance
Agency**
P.O. Box 408
One Burlington Square
Burlington, VT 05402–0408
802/864–5743

**Virgin Islands Housing
Finance Authority**
5–6 Kogens Gade
P.O. Box 12029
St. Thomas, VI 00801
809/774–4481

**Virginia Housing
Development Authority**
601 South Belvidere
Richmond, VA 23220–6504
804/782–1986

**Washington State Housing
Finance Commission**
1111 3rd Avenue, Suite 2240
Seattle, WA 98101–3202
206/464–7139

**West Virginia Housing
Development Fund**
814 Virginia Street, East
Charleston, WV 25301
304/345–6475

**Wisconsin Housing &
Economic Development
Authority**
P.O. Box 1728
Madison, WI 53701–1728
608/266–2893

**Wyoming Community
Development Authority**
P.O. Box 634
Casper, WY 82602
307/265–0603

Appendix III: General Resources

Organizations and Agencies

Action
806 Connecticut Avenue NW
Washington, DC 20525

Administration on Aging
 (AoA)
U.S. Dept. of Health and
 Human Services
330 Independence Avenue SW
Washington, DC 20201

Aging Network Services
Suite 907
4400 East-West Highway
Bethesda, MD 20814

American Association of
 Homes for the Aging
 (AAHA)
and **Continuing Care**
 Accreditation Commission
 (CCAC)
1129 20 Street NW
Suite 400
Washington, DC 20036

American Association of
 Retired Persons (AARP)
1909 K Street NW
Washington, DC 20049

American Health Care
 Association
1201 L Street NW
Washington, DC 20005

Commission on Legal
 Problems of the Elderly
American Bar Association
1800 M Street NW
Washington, DC 20036

Consumer Information Center
P. O. Box 100
Pueblo, CO 81009

Consumer Product Safety
 Commission,
 Office of Information
 & Public Affairs
5401 Westbard Avenue
Bethesda, MD 20207

Council of State Housing Agencies
400 N. Capital Street NW
Suite 291
Washington, DC 20001

Elder Craftsmen
135 East 65 Street
New York, NY 10021

Elderhostel
Suite 400
80 Boylston Street
Boston, MA 02116

Farmers Home Administration (FmHA)
South Agriculture Building
14 Street & Independence
  Avenue SW
Washington, DC 20250

Gray Panthers
Suite 601
311 South Juniper Street
Philadelphia, PA 19107

Institute for Consumer Policy Research
256 Washington Street
Mt. Vernon, NY 10553

Life Safety Systems, Inc.
2100 M Street NW
#305
Washington, DC 20037

Manufactured Housing Institute, Public Affairs Dept.
1745 Jefferson Davis Highway
Arlington, VA 22202

Medic Alert Foundation
P. O. Box 1009
Turlock, CA 95381

National Action Forum for Midlife and Older Women
c/o Dr. Jane Porcino
P.O. Box 816
Stony Brook, NY 11790

National Alliance of Senior Citizens
2525 Wilson Boulevard
Arlington, VA 22201

National Association of Area Agencies on Aging (N4A) and **National Association of State Units on Aging (NASUA)**
600 Maryland Avenue SW
Suite 208
Washington, DC 20024

National Association for Home Care
519 C Street NE
Washington, DC 20002

National Association of Housing and Redevelopment Officials
2600 Virginia Avenue
Washington, DC 20037

National Association of
  Private Geriatric Care
  Managers
1315 Talbott Tower
Dayton, OH 45402

National Center for Home
  Equity Conversion
1210 East College Drive
Suite 300
Marshall, MN 56258

National Consumers League
1522 C Street NW
Suite 406
Washington, DC 20005

National Council of Senior
  Citizens
925 15 Street NW
Washington, DC 20005

National Council on the
  Aging (NCOA)
600 Maryland Avenue SW
West Wing 100
Washington, DC 20024

National HomeCaring
  Council
235 Park Avenue South
New York, NY 10003

National Institute on Adult
  Day Care
Dept. P, 600 Maryland
  Avenue SW
West Wing 100
Washington, DC 20024

National Institute on Aging,
  Public Information Office
9000 Rockville Pike
Building 31, Room 5C35
Bethesda, MD 20892

National League for Nursing/
  American Public Health
  Association
10 Columbus Circle
New York, NY 10019

National Policy Center on
  Housing and Living
  Arrangements for Older
  Americans, University of
  Michigan
200 Bonistrel Boulevard
Ann Arbor, MI 48109

National Safety Council
444 North Michigan Avenue
Chicago, IL 60611

National Senior Citizens Law
  Center
Suite 400
2025 M Street NW
Washington, DC 20036

National Shared Housing
  Resource
6344 Greene Street
Philadelphia, PA 19144

Older Women's League (OWL)
Suite 300
730 11 Street NW
Washington, DC 20001

Share-A-Home Associations
701 Driver Avenue
Winter Park, FL 32789

Volunteers of America
3813 North Causeway
Boulevard
Metairie, LA 70002

Selected Readings*

General

American Association of Retired Persons (AARP). *Housing Options for Older Americans.* Washington, D.C.: AARP, 1985.

————. *Understanding Senior Housing for the 1990s: An American Association of Retired Persons Survey of Consumer Preferences, Concerns, and Needs.* Washington, D.C.: AARP, 1990.

————. *Your Home, Your Choice.* Washington, D.C.: AARP, in cooperation with the Federal Trade Commission, 1985. (Publication no. D12143.)

Carlin, Vivian F., and Ruth Mansberg. *Where Can Mom Live? A Family Guide to Living Arrangements for Older Parents.* Lexington, Mass.: Lexington Books, 1987.

Hancock, Judith Ann. *Housing for the Elderly.* New Brunswick, N.J.: Center for Urban Policy Research, 1987.

National Council of Jewish Women, Aging Priority. *Options for Living Arrangements: Housing Alternatives for the Elderly.* 1980. (Available through National Council of Jewish Women, Aging Priority, 12 East 26 Street, New York, N.Y. 10010.)

Sumichrast, Michael, Ronald G. Shafer, and Marilyn Sumichrast. *Planning Your Retirement Housing.* Glenview, Ill.: Scott, Foresman & Co., 1984. (An AARP book.)

Urban Land Institute. *Housing for a Maturing Population.* Washington, D.C.: Urban Land Institute, 1988.

Chapter 2

New Jersey Department of Community Affairs (NJDCA). *Home Equity Conversion Study.* Trenton, N.J.: NJDCA Task Force on Housing Options for Senior Citizens, January 1988.

Scholen, Ken. *Home-Made Money: A Consumer's Guide to Home Equity Conversion.* 2d ed. Washington, D.C.: AARP, Consumer Affairs, Program Department, 1990.

*To order copies of AARP materials, write to: AARP Publications, Program Resources Dept/BV, 1909 "K" Street NW, Washington, DC 20049.

Chapter 3

American Association of Retired Persons (AARP). *CHISS: Consumer's Guide on Accessory Apartments*. Washington, D.C.: AARP, 1987.

————. *CHISS: Consumer's Guide to Home Sharing*. Washington, D.C.: AARP, 1987 (Publication no. D12774).

————. *Legal Issues: Accessory Apartments—Zoning Covenants Restricting Land to Residential Uses*. Washington, D.C.: AARP, 1985. (Publication no. D1188.)

Dobkin, Leah. *Shared Housing for Older People: A Planning Manual for Match-up Programs*. Philadelphia: Shared Housing Resource Center, 1983.

Hare, P. H. *Creating an Accessory Apartment*. New York: McGraw-Hill, 1986.

Hare, P. H., and S. Dwight. *Accessory Apartments: Using Surplus Space in Single Family Houses*. Chicago: American Planning Association, 1981.

Murray, Priscilla. *Shared Homes: A Housing Option for Older People*. Washington, D.C.: International Center for Social Gerontology, 1975.

Shared Housing Resource Center. *Is Homesharing for You? A Self-Help Guide for Homeowners and Renters*. Philadelphia: Shared Housing Resource Center, 1983.

————. *National Directory of Shared Housing Programs for Older People*. Philadelphia: Shared Housing Resource Center, 1983.

Chapter 5

A Consumers' Guide to Home Adaptation. Boston, Mass.: Adaptive Environments Center, June 1989. (A copy may be obtained for $1.00. Send request to 621 Huntington Avenue, Boston, MA 02115.)

American Association of Retired Persons (AARP). *How to Protect Your Home*. Washington, D.C.: AARP, 1982.

LaBuda, Dennis R., ed. *The Gadget Book: Ingenious Devices for Easier Living*. Glenview, Ill.: AARP, 1985.

Raschko, Bettyann B. *Housing Interiors for the Disabled and Elderly*. New York: Van Nostrand Reinhold, 1982.

Salmen, John P. S. *The Do-Able Renewable Home: Making Your Home Fit Your Needs*. Washington, D.C.: AARP, 1985.

Tools for Independent Living and Designs for Independent Living. (Write to Appliance Information Service, Whirlpool Corporation, Benton Harbor, MI 49022) 1986.

Tools for Living. (Write to 400 West Hunter Avenue, Maywood, NJ 07631.)

U.S. Consumer Product Safety Commission. *Safety for Older Consumers: Home Safety Checklist*. (A free copy is available by writing to Office of Information and Public Affairs, U.S. Consumer Product Safety Commission, Washington, D.C. 20207, or by calling 1-800-638-2772.)

Ways and Means. (Write to 28001 Citrin Drive, Romulus, MI 48174.)

Chapter 6

American Association of Retired Persons (AARP). *A Handbook About Care in the Home.* Washington, D.C.: AARP, 1989. (Publication no. D955.)

Home Care Assembly of New Jersey. *Home Health Care: A Consumer Guide.* Princeton, N.J.: Home Care Assembly of New Jersey, 1984.

National HomeCaring Council. *All About Home Care: A Consumers' Guide.* New York: National HomeCaring Council, 1983.

New Jersey Department of Community Affairs. *Federal Programs for Older Persons.* Trenton, N.J.: New Jersey Department of Community Affairs, Division on Aging, 1989.

Schwarz, Richard. "Day Care Center Brings New Perspective to Mount Vernon Elderly." *Aging* (March–April 1983), 32, 33.

U.S. Department of Health and Human Services. *Where to Turn for Help for Older Persons: A Guide for Action on Behalf of an Older Person.* Washington, D.C.: U.S. Department of Health and Human Services, Office of Human Development Services, Administration on Aging, 1987.

Chapter 7

American Association of Retired Persons (AARP). *CHISS: Local Housing Resources Guide.* Washington, D.C.: AARP, 1987. (Publication no. D12785.)

National Association of Area Agencies on Aging. *1989–90 Directory of State and Area Agencies on Aging and National Guide for Elder Care Information and Referral.* Washington, D.C.: National Association of Area Agencies on Aging, 1990.

Chapter 8

Dickinson, Peter. *Sunbelt Retirement.* New York: E. P. Dutton, 1980.

Dickinson, Peter. *Retirement Edens Outside the Sunbelt.* New York: E. P. Dutton, 1983.

Hemming, Roy, ed. *Finding the Right Place for Your Retirement.* New York: 50 Plus Guidebooks, 1983.

Howells, John. *Retirement Choices for the Time of Your Life.* San Francisco, Calif.: Gateway Books, 1987.

Institute for Consumer Policy Research. *The Older American's Guide to Housing and Living Arrangements.* Mt. Vernon, N.Y.: Institute for Consumer Policy Research, 1984.

Irwin, Robert. *The $125,000 Decision.* New York: McGraw-Hill, 1981.

Le Croissette, Dennis. *Condominium Living: Your Guide to Buying and Living in a Condominium.* Montrose, Calif.: Young-Husband Co., 1980.

Musson, Noverre. *The National Directory of Retirement Residences: Best Places to Live When You Retire.* New York: Frederick Fell, 1973.

Shattuck, Alfred. *The Greener Pastures Relocation Guide: Finding the Best States for You.* Englewood Cliffs, N.J.: Prentice-Hall, 1984.

Sumichrast, M., R. G. Shater, and M. Sumichrast. *Planning Your Retirement Housing.* Mount Prospect, Ill.: AARP/Scott, Foresman & Co., 1984.

U.S. Dept. of Housing and Urban Development, Consumer Information Center. *Questions and Answers about Condominiums: What to Ask Before You Buy.* Pueblo, Colo.: U.S. Dept. of Housing and Urban Development, Consumer Information Center, 1974.

Woodall's Retirement and Resort Communities Directory. Highland Park, Ill.: Woodalls Publishing Company, published annually.

Chapter 9

American Association of Homes for the Aging. *Continuing Care Retirement Community: A Guidebook for Consumers.* Washington, D.C.: American Association of Homes for the Aging, 1983.

Carlin, Vivian F., and Ruth Mansberg. *If I Live to Be 100: A Creative Housing Solution for Older People.* 2d ed. Princeton, N.J.: Princeton Book Co., 1989.

————. *Where Can Mom Live? A Family Guide to Living Arrangements for Older Parents.* Lexington, Mass.: Lexington Books, 1987.

National Consumers League. *A Consumer Guide to Life Care Communities.* Washington, D.C.: National Consumers League, 1985.

National Policy Center on Housing and Living Arrangements. *The Directory of Retirement Communities in the U.S.* Ann Arbor, Mich.: National Policy Center on Housing and Living Arrangements, Institute of Gerontology, University of Michigan, 1981.

Raper, Ann Trueblood, and Anne C. Kalicki, eds. *National Continuing Care Directory.* Des Plains, Ill.: Scott, Foresman & Co., 1989. (Prepared for the American Association of Homes for the Aging.)

Chapter 10

Pynoos, Jon, Evelyn Cohen, Claire Lucas, and Linda Davis. *Home Evaluation Checklist for the Elderly.* Los Angeles, Calif.: Long-Term Care Gerontology Center of UCLA/USC, 1986. (For copies, write to Assist, 8905 Fairview Road, Suite 300, Silver Spring, Md. 20910, or call (301) 589–6760.)

Pynoos, Jon, Evelyn Cohen, Claire Lucas, and Linda Davis. *Home Evaluation Resource Booklet for the Elderly.* Los Angeles, Calif.: Long-Term Care Gerontology Center of UCLA/USC, 1986. (See above for ordering information.)

Chapter 11

American Association of Retired Persons (AARP). *Introducing CHISS (Consumer Housing Information Service for Seniors).* Washington, D.C.: AARP, 1987. (Publication no. D12449.)

Fannie Mae. *A Consumer's Guide to Seniors' Housing Opportunities (SHO)*. Washington, D.C.: Fannie Mae, May 1989.

Hiatt, Lorraine G. "Smart Houses for Older People: General Considerations." *International Journal of Technology and Aging*, 1, no. 1 (Spring/Summer 1988): 11–31.

Appendix IV: Aging Services Available for Older Americans and Their Caregivers*

Area Agencies on Aging administer and support a wide range of community-based supportive and nutrition services. Because local needs differ, not all elder-care services function in the same manner or are necessarily available in every community. Services coordinated by area Agencies on Aging include access services, community-based services, in-home services, and services to residents in facilities that provide institutional long-term care. A listing of commonly available services is provided below.

| Access Services | Assisting older Americans and their caregivers with obtaining available services. |

CLIENT ASSESSMENT. Administering examinations, procedures, or tests to determine a client's need and/or eligibility for services. Information collected may include health status, financial status, daily living status, etc. Includes pre–nursing home admissions screening as well as routine health screening (blood pressure, hearing, vision, diabetes) and testing.

CARE MANAGEMENT. Review and analysis of evidence or facts concerning an individual's social, psychological, and physical health problem(s). Commonly performed to make a conclusive statement about the level of functional ability (i.e., mildly impaired, moderately impaired, severely impaired) and requisite support services needed. Usually results in a plan of care for services or assistance either in the form of a service plan or a treatment plan.

*Excerpted from: *1989–1990 Directory of State and Area Agencies on Aging*. Reprinted with permission of National Association of Area Agencies on Aging.

INFORMATION AND REFERRAL. Includes the provision of information to an individual about available public and voluntary services or resources and linkage to ensure the service will be delivered to the client. Also includes contact with the provider and/or caregivers on an individual's behalf.

TRANSPORTATION. Taking an individual from one location to another by public or personal vehicle. This may include ride-on buses or vans, or personal vehicles operated by volunteers.

Community-Based Services

Direct services available on a community level for all older Americans.

ADULT DAY CARE. A community-based group program designed to meet the needs of functionally impaired adults through an individual plan of care. It is a structured, comprehensive program that provides a variety of health, social, and related support services in a protective setting during any part of the day, but less than 24-hour care. Individuals who participate in adult day care attend on a planned basis during specified hours. Their programs vary, but services usually include counseling and health assessments, health education, personal care, therapies, nutritious midday meals, social activities, and transportation to and from the center and transportation for special outings and doctors' appointments.

CONGREGATE MEALS. Hot or cold meals that assure a minimum of one-third of the Required Daily Allowance (RDA) to a group of older persons at a group facility. Congregate meals may be made available at senior centers, schools, churches, or other sites.

LEGAL ASSISTANCE. Many communities offer legal services. For those elderly who are unable to appropriately manage their own affairs, legal and/or protective services may be needed. Such services are designed to safeguard the rights and interests of older persons, to protect them from harm, to protect their property, and to provide advice and counsel to older persons and their families in dealing with financial and business concerns. Some legal issues that older persons and their families may be interested in could include: power of attorney; guardianship; wills; "right to die" living wills; government benefits and entitlements; consumer services; landlord/tenant problems; pensions; age discrimination; family law; etc.

SENIOR CENTER PROGRAMS. Across the country, there are more than 12,000 senior centers supporting group activities for social, physical, religious, and recreational purposes. In many communities, multipurpose senior centers (MPSC) function as a focal point for comprehensive service delivery. An MPSC provides a social environment coordinating health and social services and designing adult education programs. Many centers function as meal sites and cultural centers and as such are an important vehicle for reaching the "underserved" elderly.

ELDER ABUSE PREVENTION PROGRAMS. Refers to various state and community programs such as adult protection and guardianship/conservatorship designed to alleviate situations of abuse, neglect, or self-neglect. Examples of such maltreatment could include physical abuse, psychological abuse, material abuse (theft or misuse of property), and medical abuse. All states and many local communities have an ombudsman responsible for investigating and resolving complaints made by or on behalf of residents of long-term care facilities.

EMPLOYMENT SERVICES. May include such service components as client assessment as a basis for developing a plan for securing employment; testing; job counseling and preretirement counseling; education and training; job development and job placement.

In-Home Services

Direct services to older Americans in their homes. Designed to assist individuals stay in their homes and with their families as long as possible.

HOME-DELIVERED MEALS. Often called "Meals-On-Wheels," can be delivered five or more days a week to individuals unable to shop and prepare food on their own. These services provide enhanced nutrition and a sense of security for the homebound elderly.

HOME HEALTH SERVICES. Covers many services, often under a nurse's or doctor's supervision. These may include skilled nursing care, health monitoring and evaluation, dispensing medication, physical and other types of therapy, psychological counseling, and instructing individuals or families about ongoing care.

HOMEMAKER. Assist individuals with many of the tasks essential to maintaining a household, from food shopping and preparing meals to light housekeeping and laundry.

CHORE SERVICES. Goes beyond homemaking to include more heavy-duty tasks, such as floor or window washing, minor home repairs, yardwork, and other types of home maintenance.

TELEPHONE REASSURANCE. Provided by some agencies or volunteer organizations through regular prescheduled calls to the homebound. Ensuring personal safety is the main objective of these programs, but calls also reduce social isolation by providing personal phone contact with homebound individuals.

FRIENDLY VISITING. A volunteer program of periodic neighborly visits to homebound elders for the purpose of providing social contact, interaction, and reassurance.

ENERGY ASSISTANCE AND WEATHERIZATION. Low-income home energy and weatherization assistance is available in most states to help eligible families in paying their fuel bills or weatherizing their homes (insulation, caulking, storm windows, etc.).

EMERGENCY RESPONSE SYSTEMS. Electronic devices linking an individual to a fire department, hospital, or other health facility or social service agency. Simply pressing a button triggers a communicator attached to the telephone that automatically dials the response center.

RESPITE CARE. Allows family members to take a break from their caregiving responsibilities for a short period of time.

Notes

Introduction

1. Please see Vivian F. Carlin and Ruth Mansberg, *Where Can Mom Live? A Family Guide to Living Arrangements for Elderly Parents* (Lexington, MA.: Lexington Books, 1987).
2. Ibid., 2.
3. Ibid.
4. Ibid.
5. Ibid., 3.
6. Judith D. Kasper, *Aging Alone—Profiles and Projections* (A report prepared for the Commonwealth Fund Commission on Elderly People Living Alone, Baltimore, Md., 1988), 22, 24, 25.
7. Leah Dobkin, "Innovative Housing for the Aging—A National Overview" (Paper presented at the meeting of the Northeastern Gerontological Society, May 1988).
8. Judith G. Gonyea, Robert B. Hudson, and Gary B. Seltzer, "Housing Preferences of Vulnerable Elders in Suburbia" (Paper presented at the meeting of the Gerontological Society of America, November 1989).
9. American Association of Retired Persons, *Understanding Senior Housing for the 1990s* (Washington, D.C.: AARP, 1990), 3.
10. Ibid.
11. Kasper, *Aging Alone*, 13, 16, 31.

Chapter 1

1. Excerpted from Robert L. Rubenstein, "The Home Environment of Older People: A Description of the Psychosocial Processes Linking Person to Place," *Journal of Gerontology: Social Sciences* 44, no. 2 (March 1989) S549–51. Reprinted with permission.

Chapter 2

1. Adapted from Ken Scholen, *Home-Made Money: A Consumer's Guide to Home Equity Conversion* (Washington, D.C.: AARP, 1990), 7–9. Reprinted with permission.

2. Ibid., 10.
3. Carlin and Mansberg, *Where Can Mom Live?*, 91.
4. Ibid., 96–98.
5. Scholen, *Home-Made Money,* 12–14.
6. Ibid., 15–19.
7. Ibid., 20.
8. Material obtained from Tricia Smith, "Home Equity Conversion Program" (San Francisco: CA Independent Living Resource Center, 1989).
9. Scholen, *Home-Made Money,* 24, 25.
10. Ibid., 25, 26.
11. Ibid., 32, 33.
12. Material obtained from Tom Ostrowski, mortgage loan officer, Virginia Senior Home Equity Program, Virginia Housing Development Authority, 1989.
13. Scholen, *Home-Made Money,* 34, 37.
14. Carlin and Mansberg, *Where Can Mom Live?*, 97.
15. Judith V. May, "Home Equity Conversion Mortgage Insurance Demonstration Briefing Paper" (Washington, D.C.: Office of Policy Development and Research, U.S. Department of Housing and Urban Development, September 1989).
16. Ibid.
17. Ibid.
18. "Reverse Mortgages Can Fulfill Long-Held Dreams for Elderly," *Times* (Trenton, N.J.), 5 November 1989. Reprinted with permission.
19. Ibid.

Chapter 3

1. Carlin and Mansberg, *Where Can Mom Live?*, 101.
2. Ibid., 67, 68.
3. Ibid., 68–70.
4. Ibid., 70–73.
5. Ibid., 73–74.
6. Ibid., 74–76.
7. Shared Housing Hearing held before the Subcommittee on Housing and Consumer Interests of the Select Committee on Aging, House of Representatives, 97th Congress, 1st session, 17 November 1981. (Washington, D.C.: U.S. Government Printing Office, 1982).
8. *Is Home Sharing for You? A Self-Help Guide for Homeowners and Renters* (Philadelphia: Shared Housing Resource Center, Inc., 1983).
9. Ibid.
10. Earl Gottschalk, Jr., "Doubling Up: House Sharing Rises as a Way of Beating High Prices," *Wall Street Journal,* 17 April 1981.
11. Julia Paley, "Home-Sharing Program Pairs Young and Old," *University of Pennsylvania Daily,* 8 February 1983.

12. Robert Sunley, "Home Sharing" *Proceedings—New Options for Living: Expanding Housing Choices for the Elderly* (New Jersey Department of Community Affairs, Division on Aging, September 1980, 119–24).
13. Nicholas L. Danigelis and Alfred P. Fengler, "Home Sharing: How Social Exchange Helps Elders Live at Home," *Gerontologist* 30, no. 2 (April 1990): 162–70.
14. Shared Housing Resource Center, *Is Home Sharing for You?*, 1, 3, 4. Reprinted with permission.
15. Fannie Mae, "A Consumers Guide to Seniors Housing Opportunities" (Washington, D.C.: Fannie Mae, 1989).

Chapter 4

1. Carlin and Mansberg, *Where Can Mom Live?*, 90, 94, 95.
2. Farmer's Home Administration, "Single Family Housing Loans (Section 502 Loans)" (Washington, D.C.: Farmer's Home Administration).
3. Elizabeth Phillips, "Sharp Grant Helps Residents Dull the Cold," *Catskill Mountain News* (Margretville, N.Y.), 17 April 1986.
4. John A. Krout, "Area Agencies on Aging Planning and Service Provision for the Rural Elderly. Final Report to the Retirement Research Foundation" (Fredonia, N.Y.: Suny, Fredonia, August 1989).
5. Pamphlet entitled *Volunteer Chore Program,* published by Catholic Community Services, Tacoma, Washington.

Chapter 5

1. "Senior Citizens Security Housing and Transportation Program," flyer issued by Trenton, N.J., Department of Community Affairs, Division on Aging, 1988.
2. Carlin and Mansberg, *Where Can Mom Live?*, 108–9.
3. Krout, "Rural Elderly," 81.
4. Carlin and Mansberg, *Where Can Mom Live?*, 132–34; adapted from *Safety for Older Consumers: Home Safety Checklist* (Washington, D.C.: U.S. Consumer Products Commission, June 1986).
5. Ibid., 134–35.

Chapter 6

1. Krout, "Rural Elderly," 186.
2. Carlin and Mansberg, *Where Can Mom Live?*, 103, 104.
3. *Long Term Community Care,* brochure published by Trenton, N.J., Mercer Street Friends Center.

4. Ruth Von Behren, "Adult Day Care: A Decade of Growth," *Prospective on Aging* (July–August 1989): 14.
5. Carlin and Mansberg, *Where Can Mom Live?*, 102–3.

Chapter 7

1. John E. Hanson, "From the Publisher's Desk," *Aging Network News,* September 1989.
2. National Association of Geriatric Care Managers, *What Is a Private Geriatric Care Manager?* (Dayton, Oh.: National Association of Private Geriatric Care Managers), 1.
3. Carlin and Mansberg, *Where Can Mom Live?*, 91–93.

Chapter 8

1. Glenn Collins, "Increasing Number of Aged Return North from Florida," *New York Times,* 15 March 1984.
2. "Sunbelt Update: Older Americans," *American Demographics,* December 1984.

Chapter 9

1. Most of this chapter is based on material from Carlin and Mansberg, *Where Can Mom Live?*, chapters 2, 3, 4, 6.

Chapter 10

1. Carlin and Mansberg, *Where Can Mom Live?*, chapter 7.

Chapter 11

1. "Products and Services," *Spectrum,* March–April 1989, 25.
2. Ibid.
3. Lorraine G. Hiatt, "Understanding the Physical Environment," *Pride Institute Journal of Long-Term Care* 4, no. 2 (1985): 15.
4. Ibid., 16.
5. Lorraine G. Hiatt, "Smart Houses for Older People: General Considerations," *International Journal of Technology and Aging* 1, no. 1 (Spring–Summer 1988): 11–30.
6. "The Home Repairs for Older Americans and Disabled Homeowners Act of 1990" (introduced in the U.S. House of Representatives on 31 January 1990).

7. Dr. Robert W. Taylor, "Voluntary Rent Control and Aging in Place," Upper Montclair State College Urban Studies Program, Upper Montclair, N.J., 1988.

8. "A Consumer's Guide to Seniors' Housing Opportunities (SHO)" (Washington, D.C.: Fannie Mae, May 1989).

9. Numbers for Fannie Mae Regional offices: Southeastern area, (404) 365–6129; Southwestern area, (214) 770–7345 or 7338; Northeastern area, (215) 574–1411 or 1419 or 1440; Midwestern area, (312) 368–6279 or 6280; Western area, (818) 568–5140.

10. David Telson, ed., *Aging in Place: Supporting the Frail Elderly in Residential Environments* (Glenview, Ill.: Scott, Foresman & Co., 1990), 233.

11. This idea was presented in a paper as part of plenary Session 2, "Aging in Place," at the American Society of Aging's Annual Conference held in Washington, D.C., March 1989.

12. Russell W. Heresford, "Developing Nontraditional Home-Based Services for the Elderly," *ORB,* March 1989, 92–97.

13. Victoria Weisfeld, Terrance Keenan, and Stephen A. Somers, "Life Care at Home: New Options for the Elderly," *Aging Network News 5,* no. 1 (May 1988): 1, 16.

14. Paper written by Donald L. Moon, president, Jeanes/Foulkeways Corporation, Philadelphia, PA, 1989.

15. These stories are taken from several recent issues of *Life Care Lives,* a publication of Jeanes/Foulkeways Life Care at Home Plan, Philadelphia.

16. "Employers and Eldercare," *Working Age* (AARP Newsletter) 4, no. 6 (May–June 1989): 3.

17. CHISS Information Pak, CHISS Consumer Affairs, Program Department, AARP, Washington, D.C., 1989.

Index

About the
Author

Vivian F. Carlin received a Ph.D. in social policy and gerontology from Rutgers University. Also a certified psychologist, Dr. Carlin is a consulting gerontologist who specializes in housing and preretirement planning. Coauthor of *If I Live to be 100 . . . A Creative Housing Solution for Older People* and *Where Can Mom Live? A Family Guide to Living Arrangements for Older Parents,* Dr. Carlin retired from her position as supervisor of the Office of Planning and Policy Analysis of the New Jersey State Division on Aging. On the division staff for fifteen years, she developed such new programs as Elderly Home Conversion (the first in the U.S.) and Congregate Housing Services (the first in New Jersey and third in the nation). She has presented papers and led training sessions at regional, national, and international gerontology conferences, and has appeared as a guest on a number of radio and TV shows.